THERE
IS AN
ANSWER

Esperanza Series

THERE IS AN ANSWER

How to Prevent and Understand HIV/AIDS

The Reverend Luis Cortés Jr.

ATRIA BOOKS

New York London Toronto Sydney

ATRIA BOOKS

1230 Avenue of the Americas
New York, NY 10020

Library of Congress Catologing-in-Publicaton Data

Cortés, Luis, Reverend.
  There is an answer : how to prevent and understand HIV/AIDS / Luis Cortés
    p. cm. — (Esperanza series)
  Includes bibliographical references.
   1. AIDS (Disease) 2. AIDS (Disease)—Prevention. 3. AIDS (Disese)—Religious
aspects—Christianity. I. Title. II. Series.

RA643.8C67 2006
616.97'92—dc22   2006048352

IBN-13:   978-0-7432-8987-0
ISBN-10:   0-7432-8987-0

First Atria Books trade paperback edition October 2006

10 9 8 7 6 5 4 3 2 1

ATRIA BOOKS is a trademark of Simon & Schuster, Inc.

Manufactured in the United States of America

For information regarding special discounts for bulk purchases,
please contact Simon & Schuster Special Sales at 1-800-456-6798
or business@simonandschuster.com.

CONTENTS

Introduction   *vii*

PART 1

Diagnosis Confirmed   *1*

HIV/AIDS Can Affect Anyone   *9*

PART 2

A Family in Trouble   *15*

The Global Reach of HIV/AIDS   *20*

The New Trouble Spots   *20*

The Reported Successes   *23*

Some Sobering Realities   *26*

PART 3

Working It Out   31

Responses to HIV/AIDS: Making Progress   37

PART 4

False Comfort   47

A Pastoral Perspective   49

PART 5

More Bad News   55

Becoming Part of the Solution   62

What Can *I* Personally Do?   66

For (Brave) Men Only   68

PART 6

The Final Hours   73

A Letter from Marcus   81

Epilogue   85

Acknowledgments   89

Appendix: Helpful Organizations
   Throughout the United States   91

Sources Cited   131

INTRODUCTION

Let's play a game. I'll give you a word, and you associate it with the first thing that pops into your head.

"Family."

What did you think of right away? Maybe you had a flash of good memories and comfort. Maybe you said "food" or "happy" or "love." On the other hand, perhaps anxiety or tension was your first response: "fights," "anger," "stress." In this game, the only right answer is an honest one.

Okay, let's try another word: "friends."

Did you come up with "forever," "fun," or "good times"? Or were you having sad thoughts of loss or rejection?

One more word: "health."

"Exercise." "Vitamins." "Water." "Nutrition." "Sickness." "Doctor." Hey, you're getting good at this.

Now that we're warmed up, let's try one that's a little more difficult. What do you think of when you read "HIV/AIDS"?

Come on. Anybody? Remember, the only right answer is an honest one.

"Death." "Suffering." "Cure." "Red ribbons." "Gay." "Needles." "Africa." "I don't want to think about that."

I appreciate the last answer. That's a really honest one. Why think about something so devastating when you can't do anything about it, anyway? In fact, most people will not take an interest in this very serious subject unless a friend or family member is directly affected. That's understandable. But understand this: HIV/AIDS is in our family. Maybe it's not in your particular immediate or extended family, but it is affecting too many in our communities. No race, ethnicity, or faith is immune; the human family now suffers from HIV/AIDS.

"Well, even if it is closer to home than I thought," you might say, "what can I do about it?" There is something—there are a few important things, in fact—that you personally can do. Even if you are not a doctor, a politician, a minister, or a friend or relative of someone who is facing this disease, you can help build the firewall against HIV/AIDS, and build a more welcoming world for those who are already directly affected by it.

I just want to give you the straight deal on what's happening in the world, and in our communities, with HIV/AIDS these days. We have known about the virus—HIV—for twenty-five years. Smart, caring people have been working on the problem for about that long. It's still a serious problem, but now we have treatments and many more ways of getting care to people, even to those who are poorest and hardest to reach in the world. The best success story is this: the ranks of smart, caring people are growing. That's because people like you, who might once have believed there was no point in thinking about HIV/AIDS, are now thinking, learning, and telling others what they know.

I'm no medical expert. Nor did I write this book as someone discussing a virus called HIV. I wrote it as a man concerned about his community. In our work in community development—building homes, schools, job training centers, and health centers—we have learned a lot about the impact one person can have on a family, a neighborhood, a city, or the world.

To help you better understand some of the information provided in this book, we present the story of Marc and Delia, a married couple whose lives, along with the lives of their entire family, are irrevocably changed by the presence of HIV/AIDS. Please note that Marc, Delia, and the family members and friends in this book are *fictional*; however, their tragedy is all too real for the millions of people who live with HIV/AIDS in the family. As you read Marc and Delia's story, it is extremely important for you to ignore the fact that they are characters, and accept what they *represent*. They could be people you know—family members, friends, neighbors, coworkers. The young man who packs your groceries into a bag at the supermarket; the elderly woman you see on the bus as you go to work every day; the child who attends school with your son or daughter.

Sadly, how our imaginary family deals with Marc and Delia's awful circumstances can also be considered fictional in most cases. However, it does represent hope—hope for what our real-life community *could* become if people didn't give in to fear, pride, and deafening silence. The purpose of our story is not to scare you or suggest to you that the problem of HIV/AIDS has become hopeless. The purpose is to help us first acknowledge that there *is* a problem, because by doing so, we move much closer to a solution.

Hay una respuesta—there is an answer. And that answer begins with *you.*

I invite you to go at any time to our website, www.esperanza.us, for more information about HIV/AIDS and what you can do to fight it. I also invite you to join thousands of others who have taken the *Pacto*—the Esperanza pledge.

—The Reverend Luis Cortés Jr.

PART 1

Diagnosis Confirmed

He hadn't heard the receptionist the first two times she called him; his thoughts were someplace other than the doctor's waiting room. When she finally got his attention, she was mispronouncing his name.

"Mr. San Ray-feel."

Marc hesitated before standing up. He was fighting the feeling that when she had called him earlier—when he hadn't been paying attention—maybe she had said or done something to hint at the reason for his visit. From his seat in the far corner of the room, he had to walk toward the doctor's office in front of about twenty pairs of eyes. Dr. Gabriel was a specialist in infectious diseases who handled many kinds of conditions, but he was famous for treating AIDS patients. *The others in the room will know about me*, Marc thought nervously; then he forced himself to cross the floor calmly.

The idea that the waiting area might be filled with people facing the same trouble that he was did not occur to him until he was sitting alone in the examination room. He leaned his head against the wall and waited for the doctor. *Maybe the first test was wrong*, he told himself, *a cruel joke or mistake somehow. I could sue. God, please let it be a mistake. Come on, God. I haven't been a bad person. Let me off this one time. . . .*

Dr. Gabriel looked over the file the nurse had left for him—Marcus San Rafael, initial positive for HIV, overall health good.

"Married," the doctor said softly to himself. This diagnosis was never easy to deliver. People still heard a diagnosis of HIV-positive as a death sentence, even with treatment available. Some got angry. Some became so distraught they thought of killing themselves, rather than face the suffering they believed was inevitable.

When you told people they were HIV-positive, of course, you also had to instruct them to inform any of their sexual partners, or to give the authorities as much information as possible so that people could be contacted and informed within a few weeks. The doctor was usually able to keep the initial consultation cut-and-dried and let the patient process his or her personal issues over the course of a few weeks. Even those with live-in partners usually took a little mental and emotional time for themselves, to assess their own condition before confronting the suffering it might bring to the lives of others.

For all infected individuals, a meteor shower of fears assembled instantly and came hurtling at them all at once—the fear of their own suffering and death, the fear that people they loved would leave or be taken from them, the fear that they had already made someone else sick, the fear that their financial situation would become impossible. Many of their fears they couldn't name, but often they still tried to deal with all of them at once.

Dr. Gabriel took a deep breath as he entered the room. "Hello, Mr. San Rafael," he said, positive and businesslike, keeping his eyes on the chart that he had already memorized. "How are you today?"

"I guess you'll tell me," Marc said, trying to be light and casual.

"Well, let's see. You've tested positive for human immunodeficiency virus, and your follow-up test confirms these results. So, we're here today to talk about care for you."

Marc was only half-listening to the doctor. His thoughts careened and bounced off one another like bumper cars at the amusement park. *Oh, no. Hold on, dude—no crying, no screaming. But I want to do both. What am I going to do? I feel like I am going to throw up. The doctor is there looking at his damn chart, waiting for me to say something. Say something to the doctor, Marcus, say something.*

"Wait, hold up. You mean I have AIDS?" he blurted out.

"No, Mr. San Rafael, you have had two positive tests for the human immunodeficiency virus—HIV. The second test is fairly detailed and very reliable. It just shows that the virus is present in your body, and in enough quantity to be of concern.

"It is true that HIV can become AIDS," the doctor added. "If your immune system is disabled by the virus to the point where you contract two or more illnesses that your body can't fight— what we call opportunistic infections—you will be considered to have AIDS. But it is also true that there is treatment available that can prevent that from happening."

"But, Doctor, I don't understand. If I have this, why don't I feel sick?"

"A virus is a living organism, but HIV is a retrovirus. It can't live on its own. It must connect to the genetic material in white blood cells in order to live and multiply. Once it is inside, it starts destroying your white blood cells. The more your white blood cell count is reduced, the harder it is for your body to fight other viruses, bacteria, or fungi that produce disease. Unless or until your immune system is severely weakened, you may not have symptoms. You may not even feel sick."

"When *will* I feel it?" Marc asked, still clearly in shock.

"When we evaluate a patient's progress with the virus, we look at the count of a certain type of white blood cell that we call CD4. The average healthy person has a CD4 count of 700 to 1,200. We become concerned when the level drops to half the normal immune level, but even at 350, people can still be doing well. It's possible that at some point you may develop flulike symptoms. We usually don't begin treatment with antiretroviral drugs until the count reaches 200 or lower, but the option is available once you hit 350."

"So, you'll give me medicine and I'll get better?"

"We would not start you on medication yet," Dr. Gabriel answered. "The medications we have so far are effective at slowing the progress of HIV, but they can bring about serious side effects. We have to weigh the benefits against the potential risks, so we generally prescribe them only when the immune system is severely debilitated. Your white blood cell count is still fairly high—around 500."

"But I read the other day that someone discovered a cure."

"Recently, there has been some encouraging research, but it was very limited. Those discoveries will have to be tested over and over again before anything useful can be developed."

"Okay. So, what do I do now?" Marc asked the doctor, then realized he was also asking himself. *What do I do now? Delia, the kids, my job, Abuela . . . everybody will run from me. No one must know.*

"We will do a lifestyle assessment to see if you are in any one of several risk categories. If your risk level is limited, we would monitor your CD4 count every six months. We could also monitor what is called your viral load—how much virus is in your body.

"Our nurse-practitioner can give you detailed counsel about how to take care of your health so that you can keep your immunity boosted, avoid infections, and give yourself the best chance of keeping your count up. Of course, if you notice any change in your health, we'll want you to contact us before your six-month test."

"How did I get it? I thought you had to be gay or shooting drugs to get AIDS."

"Again, Mr. San Rafael, you don't have AIDS," Dr. Gabriel reiterated. "You have had a confirmed positive result in a test for HIV. HIV transmission is complex, but if you have the patience, I will tell you a little about what we know at this point. It is possible to transmit the virus during intercourse between a man and a woman. There are other ways, of course—unprotected sex is the main way; and, as you noted, the use of infected needles is also a major way.

"We have identified certain conditions that are either more or less favorable to transmission. Some of these have to do with the pH of the body fluids in question—fluids such as blood or semen are good environments for the virus. Saliva and acidic media, such as urine, are less hospitable. The virus is not transmitted through the air, from things like a sneeze or cough. We don't know yet whether one exposure is enough for transmission, but common sense would certainly suggest that the more often someone is exposed to the virus under conditions in which it can survive, the more chances there are for transmission."

"So, my kids can't get it?"

"Most children who are HIV-positive contract the virus in the womb or during birth from an HIV-positive mother. Of course, children, like all people, do become at risk if they are exposed to infected needles or blood products, or if they come into sexual contact with a person carrying the virus.

"One precaution I would suggest in your household would be to carefully guard items used for shaving. Also, take extra care with open wounds. And I can't emphasize enough that you should encourage your wife to be tested immediately, so she can be cared for as well, and so we can determine any possibility that the virus has been transmitted to one of your children."

Marc was silent for a while, trying to take in all this information. Finally he looked at the doctor. "What about my wife?" he asked quietly.

"She will absolutely need to be tested. So will anyone else you may have had sexual relations with in the last few years."

Marc stared at the floor. "But is she going to get it?"

"There are three possibilities. One possibility is that because you now know, you will take every precaution and she will not contract the virus. The second possibility is that she may already have contracted it from you. Or, third, you may have contracted it from her."

Noticing the sudden glare from Marc, the doctor paused briefly and looked away. "In any event," he continued, "it is best for her that she be tested immediately. You can make an appointment for her before you leave if you like, and I'll give you some more information which you can share with her."

Marc thanked Dr. Gabriel. It felt a little odd, thanking someone for shattering his life, but he shook the doctor's hand and left the examination room. He didn't notice the faces of anyone he passed by on his way out the door and onto the street. He headed home with the face of only one person on his mind: his wife, Delia. It would be their wedding anniversary in two days.

* * *

I don't like HIV, but I'm not afraid of it anymore.

I've had friends die from AIDS, but more and more, my friends who are HIV-positive are living with it, not dying from it. They're going to work, loving their families and friends, and enjoying their time on Earth. I want to be the kind of friend who lives life with them. When they need to say they're not feeling well, I want to be able to listen. When they're feeling up and ready to have fun or just be with people, I want to be able to be there.

I'm educating myself. I know you don't catch HIV from being a friend, from sharing a meal together, or from a hug. In fact, hugging your HIV-positive friend not only won't hurt you; it will probably help your friend feel better.

I'm encouraging my friends to see a doctor, to get a real diagnosis, and to get treatment. I'm encouraging them to be open with the ones they love. I'm encouraging them to come out and play on their good days, and to keep hope alive on the days that are not so good.

There are treatments. There are things people can do to maximize their health and well-being. There are caring people. There is a way to live with HIV.

There is an answer.
—José Luis Rodriguez, actor and singer

HIV/AIDS Can Affect Anyone

I'd like to present you with a typical case study of a person affected by HIV/AIDS. I'd like to, but I can't. There is no typical case. In this book, our fictional family confronts some of the issues that HIV/AIDS raises for people medically, socially, emotionally, and spiritually. We hope to illustrate how this extended family might respond in some helpful ways. This is not meant to present the perfect situation—it is meant to open up hearts and minds to more creative and compassionate responses to HIV/AIDS than we are currently seeing.

HIV stands for *human immunodeficiency virus*. This term means that if you are human, you are susceptible to it. The reality is that more people—and more kinds of people—are afflicted with and affected by HIV than ever before.

A famous American film called *Philadelphia* tells the story of Andrew Beckett, a successful attorney in the early 1980s who contracts HIV and develops AIDS—acquired immune deficiency syndrome. The large, expensive law firm where Beckett is employed tries to fire him quietly, even though his work has been superior in all respects and he is popular socially as well as professionally. He decides to risk his standing by fighting this injustice publicly. Beckett wins his court case, but ultimately loses his fight with the disease—in the story, he has developed AIDS too early in history for treatment to be available. As the virus attacks his immune system, he becomes sick with other illnesses that he cannot fight. He loses weight, loses his hair, becomes thin and gaunt, and eventually dies at the end of the film. What makes *Philadelphia* an even more moving film is that it is a true story.

There is no film, however, about the life of a young woman from San Pedro de Macorís, Dominican Republic. In her case, she can't tell her story, because she wasn't even allowed to know that she had contracted HIV. At age nineteen, pregnant, she was brought to a community health station near her home by a man who identified himself as her husband. He asked that she be tested for HIV. When her test results came back positive, he demanded that she be treated without being told why.

This man declined testing or treatment for himself, saying that he already knew he was HIV-positive and was being cared for by a private doctor in the capital city, Santo Domingo. What about his pregnant wife, the community health workers wanted to know. Why didn't he take her to his private doctor, who would certainly have access to more sophisticated care? He then admitted that she was not really his wife. His actual wife lived with him, was also HIV-positive, and was being seen by their doctor. This young woman was simply the mother of his unborn baby. He did not want the baby to become HIV-infected, so he wanted the mother to be given the treatments that would reduce the risk of her transmitting the virus to the baby. But he did not want her to know about her HIV status because then she would know about his.

The health workers were furious, arguing that it would be wrong not to inform the woman. The man became belligerent with them and said they'd better take care of his baby. He threatened them with legal action if they revealed his HIV status or that of his girlfriend to anyone, including the pregnant woman herself. Some workers from the United States at first did not believe he had legal grounds for this. Knowingly exposing your sexual partner to HIV is a crime in the United States, where laws require that prior sexual partners be informed within weeks after a person learns of an HIV infection.

Local health care workers quickly informed the U.S. workers

that Dominican laws are different. Legal officials confirmed that they could be prosecuted for libel if they gave out information about the man's HIV infection. The workers treated the woman and unborn child so as to prevent the infection from spreading further. (Medications given during pregnancy have been shown to reduce the risk of transmission from mother to child dramatically.) They did so with heavy hearts, desperate to come up with a plan that would get information to the young woman without putting her at risk of losing her only source of income—her baby's father. Adding to the heartbreak of this situation was the knowledge that the man had yet another girlfriend, to whom he had also not revealed his HIV status; nor had he taken her to a doctor. There was no need, he said, because she was not pregnant.

There *is* lots of film—news footage and public-service videos—about the nameless multitudes of infected men, women, and children in Africa, where the first documented HIV infection occurred. Africa is said to be the "ground zero" of AIDS; of the tens of millions worldwide who have died since the start of the epidemic, almost one-third of them—roughly 25 million—have been in southern Africa. In some villages throughout this area, AIDS has taken the life of every adult, leaving children to raise themselves as well as younger brothers and sisters.

In one such tragedy, the parents of a family of six children died. The oldest brother, seeing his parents' fate, had the presence of mind to seek out health care workers and beg for testing and treatment. He was found to be HIV-positive, with a quickly progressing case of AIDS. Treatment did not save him, so his next oldest brother—age nine—became the head of the household. Ten years later, that boy remains the single parent of four younger children. The family now receives assistance from a Christian relief organization.

In those ten years, progress has been made in developing treatment, preventing transmission, and getting care to people who need it. There still is a lot of work to do, but today it is fueled with a lot more hope.

One puzzle the smart and caring people of the world are currently working to solve is that even with all the information and treatment available today, one-third to one-half of people who carry HIV don't even know it. In lower-income communities throughout the United States, 35 to 40 percent of people who should be tested are not. In third world countries, more than half of those with HIV remain unaware of it. And among those who do know their status, very few get complete care.

Esperanza USA and the groups with which we work are trying to do our part. In 1987, we supported the establishment of a full-service health clinic in inner-city Philadelphia. Clinic services include HIV testing, counseling, and ongoing care. We also have partnered with Sembrando Flores, founded and directed by Nancy Rivera in Miami; Bruised Reed Ministry, founded and directed by Reverend Rosa Caraballo in New York City; and Access Caribe in the Dominican Republic. These faith-based groups have concerned themselves with meeting the needs of the whole person—income assistance, housing, family counseling and support, and end-of-life care. They have also made it clear that all are welcome, embracing fully those who bear the extra burden of HIV/AIDS in the family. Today Esperanza USA is dedicating itself to providing tools that will help educate our Hispanic community—as well as everyone else—about this epidemic. To this end, we have produced music, films, and written resources, all of which you can learn more about at www.esperanza.us.

The former medical director of the Esperanza Health Clinic in Philadelphia—Dr. Ramón Gadea, who is a specialist in infectious diseases—has gone on to found Access Caribe, through which he, fellow medical professionals, and volunteers are working to establish clinics that provide HIV care in the Dominican Republic. They too are finding that sometimes the best way to get care to people with HIV is to offer assistance with a full range of needs. Prenatal care, maternity care, and community visits to provide health care and screenings are just three examples of the ways in which Access has been able to reach people who might not have seen a doctor otherwise.

There is no "typical" HIV/AIDS case. Therefore, there is no typical response to HIV/AIDS. People who receive the diagnosis go through the stages of grief—shock and denial, anger, bargaining, depression, and acceptance—as do the people who love them. However, as we have stated and will continue to emphasize, a positive test for HIV is *not* a death sentence. There is still life to live, and there are choices to make about which friends and family one brings into the circle of support.

Dr. Gadea has commented that with advances in research, sometimes the medical aspect of caring for someone with HIV/AIDS is the easiest part. He has also observed that in the Hispanic community, when people have gotten past the thick, high wall of secrecy and told trusted individuals what's happening in their lives, other, more positive values in our culture present themselves: family ties, a sense of community, and deep and long-standing spiritual values.

Right now, the numbers are discouraging for the worldwide Hispanic community. Roughly one-fourth of newly diagnosed pediatric AIDS cases are Hispanic children. AIDS has become the fourth leading cause of death for Hispanic women under age fifty, and the second leading cause of death for Hispanic men under fifty.

Our community can rally, however. The work of Nancy Rivera, Rosa Caraballo, and Ramón Gadea illustrates this fact. In the Appendix of this book, you will find a list of many more organizations working among Hispanic people to decrease the spread of HIV/AIDS.

Recent figures show that there are 750,000 AIDS orphans in Latin America. For the most part, these children have been taken into the homes of neighbors or members of the extended family, so there has not yet been any large-scale movement in Latin America to open AIDS orphanages. Let's do our part—while we can—to make sure there is never a need to do so.

PART 2

A Family in Trouble

Dr. Gabriel had said that Marc should tell his wife right away. She had a right to know.

That had made sense in Dr. Gabriel's office, but standing here at his own front door, Marc was afraid all over again. He hoped that she wasn't home. That maybe he could just take a few minutes to go in, take his shoes off, sit down, and watch TV for a while.

But no sooner had he entered the bedroom to change his clothes than he heard Delia walk in the front door.

"Hi, honey, you're home early," she said, giving him a quizzical look and a peck on the cheek.

He had never been so scared in his life. He finished hanging his work clothes on the peg behind the bedroom door, and then turned to her. He had never been good at hiding his feelings, and he knew from the look on Delia's face, before he even said anything, that she realized something bad was happening.

"Marc, what's going on? What's wrong? Why are you home early? Why are you so quiet? Did you get laid off? What happened?"

"Delia . . . *mami.*" The words stuck in his throat. "I have to tell you something."

She had sat in the closet for hours. "I need to be alone. I need to think," she had said. "What did you do?" she screamed at one point. "What did you do? *¿Qué porquería?*"

"Delia, baby, please—"

"Marc, go downstairs!" she shouted. "Get out! I can't talk to you now. I know I will have to talk to you, but not now. Tomorrow. Go away. *¡Ay, señor!*"

She started crying again.

It was a long night. Marc had told the kids to make some food for themselves and then come kiss him good night. Mommy wasn't feeling well, he said. He was going to stay up for a little while, give Mommy a chance to rest, and then check on her.

He lay down on the couch and watched TV. He slept a little, as the noise of infomercials played in the background. He woke up and caught a second wind at around four in the morning, so he turned the television volume up slightly.

"This village in Africa," the blonde TV actress was saying, "was once a thriving place of hunters, gatherers, and cooperative farmers. Today, it is a devastated community of homes headed by children trying to scrape out a living. A few of the frailest elders survive. HIV/AIDS is the scourge of sub-Saharan Africa, taking lives and leaving children devastated, alone, without any adults to care for them. Africa is ground zero in the HIV/AIDS pandemic. But, thank God, there is hope. . . ."

Marc suddenly realized that there were tears in his eyes. He decided to just let them come. It made sense to grieve for the world, to grieve for himself. Where did this disease come from? Couldn't anybody stop it?

"Why, God?" he asked aloud. "Why me? It's unfair!"

He cried until he was exhausted, and then fell asleep just before the sun came up.

For three days Delia hadn't spoken to him. He could see that she had left snacks out for the kids for when they got home from school. But she wasn't cooking and serving dinner; in fact, she wouldn't even come out of the bedroom if he was home.

Marc would pick up dinner on the way home from work. "Mommy's still not feeling well. She needs to rest," was all he would tell the kids. Finally, his sister-in-law suggested, "Bring the kids to me for a few days. Let her work through it, Marcus. It's a shock, you know?"

Once they left, Delia left, too. She went to stay with a friend who lived closer to her job. At least that's what he guessed from the scribbles on the little pad near the telephone in the kitchen.

Marc was alone. Having the place to himself used to be nice, when he knew they were coming back—from a game after school or from the supermarket, where the three of them stopped sometimes after Delia met the kids at the bus stop on her way home from work.

She worked so hard, and had done so all her life. She had wanted more kids than the two they had, but Marc had been so sure they couldn't afford it. He had worked hard, too, and he had wanted them to live at least a little better than both their parents had. They had gotten a little closer to their dreams—they were only a couple of years away from being able to buy a small house. Lately, Delia had even allowed herself to fantasize a little. He had caught her looking at furniture ads in the newspaper, drawing little pictures, and filling in colors with the kids' crayons.

There was no reason not to cry. No one was there to see. He leaned against the kitchen wall, near the phone, and sobbed. His knees gave out, so he just sat on the kitchen floor and cried. "God, please," he begged, "I'll do anything. Change this, please."

Marc didn't move for hours. It grew dark outside, and soon the only light in the kitchen came from the small night-light plugged into the outlet near the stove. He curled up on the floor and fell asleep.

*   *   *

It's true that Latin America doesn't have an AIDS crisis like the one we've seen in Africa. But it's not true that the Latin world doesn't have an AIDS problem.

We have a chance to win this struggle, but at the moment we are playing catch-up. Why? Because, surveys show, Latinos do not like to talk about HIV/AIDS.

No one likes to talk about AIDS, but with 1.7 million people in Latin America living with HIV, with almost 100,000 deaths last year, and with a rising infection rate among Latin women and children in the United States, there is a lot to talk about.

There are already over 350,000 AIDS orphans in Las Americas, with the Dominican Republic alone having 50,000. Let's not see any more.

So much is now available to us: new medicines, more precise testing, community health projects, and better information. We have a chance to beat this in our communities throughout the United States and Latin America. But first we have to talk.

There is an answer.

— Ricardo Montaner, singer

The Global Reach of HIV/AIDS

Only one continent in the world has no problem with AIDS: Antarctica. Meanwhile, Africa, where the first human infection is believed to have occurred, has had the greatest number of deaths, has the highest rates of infection, and has some of the most complicated social issues to unravel. Southern Africans still make up one-third of the world's AIDS cases, though the latest figures from the United Nations show encouraging progress in the nations of Kenya, Uganda, and Lesotho, where strides in prevention and containment have been made.

After Africa, the region most affected by AIDS will be either India or the Caribbean—at present, this is a toss-up. Those who monitor the pandemic full-time predict that India and its surrounding regions will eventually follow Africa in sheer numbers of infections and deaths. At the moment, however, the nations of the Caribbean basin are far in the lead, in terms of the percentage of the population that is affected and the rate at which infection is occurring. Still, the latest figures from the United Nations are encouraging: while the percentages of those infected are still high, the Caribbean is the one area in the world where the incidence of HIV/AIDS did not increase in the past year.

The New Trouble Spots

The Indian peninsula is blinking steadily on the radar screens of people keeping track of the AIDS pandemic. One of the measures that these AIDS-watchers use is based on the percentage of the population that is HIV-positive. In India, less than 1 percent of the overall population is affected. However, another measure used is based on the actual numbers of people who are HIV-positive, have AIDS, or have died from AIDS. These numbers for India and its surrounding regions are approaching levels that were last seen in Africa, when the crisis was first emerging on that continent.

To date, six states in the nation of India have broken the 1 percent barrier. In these states more than 1 percent of the population is HIV-positive. When 1 percent or more of the people in a nation or region are infected, that area is considered to have an epidemic.

AIDS-watchers are worried about these areas in India as well as nearby areas of Bangladesh and Pakistan because, like the crisis areas throughout Africa, these regions also have other social problems to battle—poverty, poor public sanitation, and limited health and nutrition resources. In these regions, unlike in Africa, population density is quite uniformly high. History and common sense teach that it is harder to contain the spread of an infectious disease—even a disease that is not airborne—when large numbers of people live in close quarters throughout an impoverished region.

The Caribbean is of even greater concern for AIDS-watchers. There were roughly 1,000 deaths per day in 2004, and then the number dropped to about 24,000 for all of 2005. These figures do not sound high compared with those from sub-Saharan Africa, but the Caribbean includes a group of relatively small nations, and AIDS has taken over quickly in several of these countries. Remember that when more than 1 percent of the people have contracted the virus, an epidemic is declared. The rate in the Caribbean nations was between 1 and 4 percent of the adult population infected by the end of 2005.

The numbers of men and women who are infected are equal on average, though some places have a greater infection rate in women than in men. Efforts to reach pregnant women have been fast and furious, as health care officials watched infection rates just among these women climb to between 3 and 5 percent. In the areas of greatest concern—Haiti and the Dominican Republic—these figures appear to have been brought under some control. About 1.4 percent of pregnant women in the Dominican Republic are HIV-positive; and the percentage of women in Haiti testing positive was cut in half—from 6 percent to about 3 percent. Nevertheless, these numbers are still extremely high.

Another emerging problem in addressing HIV/AIDS in the Caribbean is that it will not stay contained there. Urban centers in North America have community ties to almost every nation in the Caribbean basin, and there is regular traffic between the two areas. For every nation in the Caribbean, there is a neighborhood in New York. In the year 2000, the New York City Department of Health reported that among immigrants to the city who had HIV infection, 46 percent were from the Caribbean region, with an additional 27 percent from Latin America. In case anyone is wondering, New York does not lack immigrants from the rest of the world, but the total number of immigrants from eastern Europe, Asia, Africa, and other regions did not equal the number of HIV-positive Hispanic immigrants.

Other places—among them Jersey City, Philadelphia, and Miami—have direct links to any issues that emerge in the Caribbean countries, including, and perhaps most especially, HIV/AIDS. As Dr. Gadea, who works in both North America and the Caribbean, observed, "We are all part of the same neighborhood."

If we think that sophistication, information, and advanced medical care are the complete answer to HIV/AIDS, we are wrong:

San Juan, New York, and Los Angeles—where services and information are widely available—continually rank highest in AIDS infection rates among major North American cities.

Other regions coming up fast include China and southeast Asia; both are confronting a large and growing problem with AIDS. Russia and the Baltic states face a double threat: AIDS and a widespread outbreak of tuberculosis. Labor in this sparsely populated region of eastern Europe is so devastated that the business and industrial communities have joined forces with health officials and service organizations to find a way to stop the spread of HIV/AIDS.

North America—where the virus that causes AIDS was first discovered and documented—has had successes in delivering treatment, containing infection, and spreading the word about prevention. However, even with all the resources available and all the success, too many people still do not get care, do not understand prevention, and continue to engage in risky sexual behavior, with little regard for the very real dangers of HIV/AIDS.

The Reported Successes

- Brazil once had the dubious distinction of being home to one-third of all the people in Latin America with HIV. In its favor, it has been called a "beacon among developing countries" in implementing treatment programs. Because Brazil reportedly has been able to get retroviral medication to virtually everyone who needs and wants it, the average survival of AIDS patients has increased from five months to five years. In addition, Brazil was able to bring about a steep reduction in infections among users of intravenous drugs through the "clean needle" efforts popularized in many European countries. Sadly, though, Brazil parallels many nations in that the epidemic began among males but has leaped to the female population, whose infection rate continues to grow.

- Compared with the rest of the world, North America makes the best care available to those who are aware of their HIV status. Years ago, early organizing helped set up models in delivery of services and information. The United States was in the forefront of AIDS research, and scientists there first documented HIV as the cause of AIDS. If it were a simple matter of getting a diagnosis and getting medical care, there would be a lot less suffering in the United States than there is. It pains me to see those rising infection rates among Hispanics, African-Americans, and women and children.

- The nation of Uganda is held up as a model of success in widespread testing, public education, and delivery of treatment. Following Uganda's lead, Kenya and Lesotho have shown progress in containing the spread and broadening the treatment available.

Uganda has been successful in areas with which others are still struggling. For one thing, the whole country talks about HIV/AIDS. No one wonders what or how much to say, since Ugandans broke the "silence barrier" a long time ago. Unlike many of their neighbors, they accepted foreign help and funding, and they allowed their existing institutions to become forums for discussion and education about preventing and treating AIDS.

From what has happened in Uganda, we get an idea about what public health concerns will be in the future as understanding and action increase in other parts of the world. Uganda's current focus is to take care of the throngs of people who have now been successfully identified as HIV-infected. The successful public health campaign means that more people now know their status and presumably will take better care—not only caring for their own health but also taking care not to become a means of spreading the virus further. This is all good news in a world where the battle internationally has been to get people to admit there is a problem and allow service agencies to address it publicly. But it brings another kind of problem: getting care to everyone who is requesting it.

I have toured Africa personally, and I can assure you that any portrayal of suffering you may have seen on the news, on late-night TV infomercials, or through your association with a charitable organization or church was not exaggerated. Ignorance of what HIV/AIDS is has hurt the struggles. I was personally told numerous stories of the rapes of young women because of a myth that sex with a virgin would cure AIDS. Of course, it does not, but this myth has led to the destruction of young girls' lives and, ironically, has contributed to the spread of the disease. Throughout the world, erroneous remedies are being promoted. What we have learned is that good information, widely disseminated in a clear yet sensitive way, is crucial to health and safety.

In Africa, we have also learned that when the world cooperates we can make an incredible difference. I continue to be encouraged and inspired by the stories of wealthy and successful people who put aside the benefits of the lives they have built to go and establish outposts of relief in Africa. I am also inspired by the work done on the ground every day by people who are not celebrities and may never have their stories told, but are bringing about real, positive change here on Earth.

Some Sobering Realities

- Male homosexual intercourse remains one of the most common and most efficient means by which AIDS is transmitted. But it is not, and never was, the only means of transmission. Infected needles and sex between men and women are the other two major ways of spreading HIV. In some areas around the world, even places where AIDS has been for a long time, people still do not know these basic facts.

- In parts of Africa, surveys of women ages fifteen to twenty-four showed that these women were unaware of how AIDS is transmitted and therefore were not able to factor AIDS prevention into decisions about their lives. Women now account for 57 percent of all HIV infections in Africa.

- A study commissioned by Esperanza USA found that many Hispanic ministers and church workers still harbor the erroneous ideas that AIDS is transmitted solely through male homosexual sex and that anyone not engaged in such activity is not susceptible to the disease.

- In the Hispanic world—Latin America, the Caribbean, and the United States—the rate of female HIV infection is rising, mostly through male-female sex. In the

Caribbean, women have now achieved equal status with men, making up 49 percent of the adults there with HIV. In Latin America, the percentage is lower but rising; it is currently at 36 percent. In the United States, women account for 25 percent of adult HIV infections. Hispanic women, like Hispanic men and children, are affected in greater percentages than the general population. The AIDS case rate among Hispanic women is over five times that among Anglo women, according to the National Association of People with AIDS.

- Prostitution that serves tourists first brought the virus to Asia and parts of the Caribbean. This industry continues to thrive. The answer generally proposed in these areas, where economic vulnerability drives the continued availability of sex for sale, is to promote the demand and distribution of condoms. One report by the World Health Organization (WHO) used documented "condom sales" as a marker of success in fighting AIDS in Barbados and the Caribbean. It is true—whether or not my colleagues in the church would like to hear it—that condoms do reduce the risk of HIV transmission. But it is also true—whether or not my associates in public policy and social service agree—that abstinence outside a healthy, committed relationship works better.

- In some regions of the world—south Asia and southeast Asia, as well as parts of the Baltic states, Latin America, and Africa—there is a high volume of what is officially labeled "trafficking in children." Some of this involves farming children out to perform low-paying domestic or industrial labor. These children are at risk for all kinds of tragedy. The special tragedy of AIDS, however, is reserved for the thousands of children being forced into sex trades.

- According to one advocacy group working in India, in addition to the trauma, poverty, neglect, and abuse they had suffered, 70 percent of the girls and young women rescued from this kind of slavery were HIV-infected. People who are being forced into prostitution do not have the power to demand that customers use condoms or that "employers" provide chemical protection in the form of microbicides that, when applied before intercourse, can at least reduce the risk of HIV transmission. In some areas of southeast Asia, boys are at high risk as well because of the special demand among visitors to that region for young male prostitutes.

- One report by the United Nations estimates that 1.2 million children are sold into slave labor each year, though exact numbers are hard to obtain. Nations are understandably not proud of this, and the people running such operations keep their industry functioning through gangster-style violence against anyone who tries to interfere. Much of what is known about this situation comes through reports from aid workers and missionaries who work on the ground, in secret and at their own peril, trying to get these children free, healed, and established in a life where they can earn a living for themselves.

- In North America, we are hearing that whole segments of the population in their teens and early twenties do not take the threat of HIV/AIDS as seriously as they should, and therefore take risks with their health that could be fatal for themselves or someone else. These younger people have grown up in a world that is familiar with AIDS and have been given the facts in what advocates believed would be a style relevant to the youth culture. Yet they have turned around and adopted a "whatever" attitude about a disease that only a generation ago terrified the nation.

- We live in a world with HIV/AIDS. Not thinking about it won't make it go away, or prevent the virus from spreading. In fact, the surveys show that not thinking is one of the reasons why the virus spreads. What you don't know *can* hurt you, and it can also hurt someone else. Here is a positive fact: with so many people affected in so many areas, each of us has a great many choices these days about how to respond proactively. The only choice we really don't have is to live in a world where HIV/AIDS is not a factor . . . unless we want to move to Antarctica.

PART 3

Working It Out

For a minute, he didn't know where he was. He was stiff, cold, and a little confused. The phone was ringing. Realizing that this ringing was what had woken him, and that the sound was coming from over his head, he sat up, put his hand against the wall, and slowly pushed himself to a standing position. He didn't reach the phone before the answering machine kicked in.

"Marc," said a woman's voice. "Marc, it's Lisa."

He didn't pick up right away. He wasn't sure he could talk to anyone just then, especially his wife's closest friend.

"I wanted to get you personally, but . . ." She paused. "Listen, Marc, Delia asked me to call you. She wants to see you, Marc, but not at the house. Not where anyone can interrupt you guys or get involved in the conversation. Except she wants me to be there. I told her I would, but that you have a say in it, too. Let me know what you think, Marc. All I know is you guys have to talk. I'll do anything to help you. Call me back, okay? Dee said you two can meet at the Salvadoran place you know."

She paused again. This time Marc heard conversation in the far background.

"She said you owe her for missing your anniversary."

It felt weird, but he smiled. He almost dropped the receiver as he grabbed it off the hook.

"Lisa, it's Marc." His voice was a little hoarse, and he didn't feel he had complete control of it. "I just caught your message. I'll meet her. You can come too, if it makes her feel better. Thanks, Lisa."

Marc changed his clothes three times, but he didn't look good to himself no matter how he dressed. Junk food, worry, and lack of sleep all showed on his face. The best he could do was to put on a little of Delia's favorite cologne, and hope she wouldn't laugh at him for it.

The restaurant was close enough that he could walk. Air and exercise might steady his nerves. Why did he feel as edgy as if it were his first date? It wasn't fun like that, but it was just as scary. He was about to have to negotiate his way back into this woman's life, this woman he had been with for fifteen years.

They weren't there when he arrived. He didn't know whether to pick a table for three or two—or one. What if she changed her mind and didn't come?

The hostess approached him and started to speak, but the only voice he heard was that of his wife, now standing behind him. "Hey, Marc. Happy belated anniversary."

He wanted to grab her and squeeze her and never let her go. Instead, he just touched her face and said, "Thanks. You, too."

"Table for three?" the hostess asked.

"Yes," Delia answered as Lisa stepped up behind her.

They knew the menu, so they ordered quickly. It felt good to be doing something pleasant, familiar, and easy. Delia was actually smiling a little. Neither said much other than nice comments about the food and little updates about work. They didn't mention the kids at all.

They asked for some coffee. Marc and Delia both knew they could stay at the table until the place closed, so they waited until dessert was finished to start talking.

Delia began. She spoke softly and steadily. "I've been to the doctor. I know you thought I didn't hear you about having to get tested, but I did. You said it over and over, so how could I miss it? So I did it."

Marc froze. The noise of the plates and silverware being picked up and set down, plus the hum of conversation throughout the restaurant, blended into one steady buzz that resonated loudly in his brain. He couldn't think, much less speak, so he waited for her to continue.

"I went to the doctor, got tested, and sat with a counselor. I don't have it, Marcus. I know I'll have to go back for repeated testing, but this test was negative. I wanted Lisa to be here tonight when I told you because she made me go, honey. She made me go to the doctor. I wasn't going to—I didn't want any more bad news, you understand? But Lisa told me, 'News is news. It's not good or bad. It's just information you work with.' Well, I think she's a little wrong there. But I'm happy with the test results."

Marc jumped in. "Me, too, baby. Me, too."

"Obviously, our problems are far from over. It's just that now we have a better idea what they are. The counselor was pretty straight with me—you and I are going to have to make some pretty detailed plans about our marriage, you understand? I mean, I have every intention of being your wife, but I have every intention of staying alive long enough to be my kids' mother, too."

"Delia, I'll do whatever you say. Whatever you want, honey. I'm so happy you're not sick—"

"Marc, that's not what I need from you right now," she interrupted. "I need you to do at least half the thinking in this deal. You are the one who is going to be directly in touch with the doctors and nurses. You are going to have to keep up with what's okay and what's not okay, and not just leave it all up to me to keep things safe.

"The counselor told me to come back to see her anytime, but you and I both know that's not going to be practical forever. We have information now and we have to use it. We have to protect the kids and each other. We both have big families, jobs, church. We have to decide who needs to know and who doesn't. We have to tell the kids something, but I don't know what or when exactly. We also need some contingency plans, in case there is a rough patch when you can't work."

Delia paused momentarily, then looked directly into her husband's eyes. "Actually, there's a lot to do, so if you think I am going to come back home just to stroke your head and say, 'Poor, poor baby,' you are *so* wrong."

"But you *are* coming home?" Marc asked, trying not to hope too much.

"I want to. I want the kids to come back and for us to go about things as routinely as possible. I believe that's the best thing for us. But we have to be smart, practical, and disciplined. The counselor told me to get ready to become angry all of a sudden for no apparent reason. She said anything I'm not dealing with right now could pop up at any time—that I might become angry at you for getting sick or for the ways my imagination will tell me how you got sick.

"I know neither one of us has lived a perfect life," she continued, "but I'll need to know how and why this has happened. The counselor warned I might also shut down toward you because you have potentially burdened me with life as a single parent. Of course, she recommended love and compassion and all that. But she also said it won't do us much good to pretend all the time. Anyway, I'm talking so much and you're not saying anything. What do *you* think?"

Marc said the only thing he had wanted to say since he was first diagnosed with HIV. "I love you, honey. I am so sorry. I wanted good things for us."

"Ah, Marcus, if we're destined for good things, we'll just get to them by another road."

*　　*　　*

"AIDS was really scary in the eighties. Man, I'm glad that's over."
"AIDS is a really serious problem . . . in Africa."
"You have to be gay or shooting up to get AIDS, so I'm not worried."
"I don't feel sick. Why should I get an HIV test?"

I'm glad we can mention HIV/AIDS in public today without causing panic or hysteria. But now that we're talking, we have to get our facts straight, because people are thinking some funny things. With only about twenty years of good research behind us, it's understandable that we don't understand everything yet.

To help us all get on the same basic page, let's go over some of the things we do know for certain:

- The pandemic is not over, and it's not just in Africa. There are plenty of sick people who are neither homosexual nor using intravenous drugs. HIV can hide in your body for years without letting you know, and you can infect someone else even if you don't feel sick.

- If you have ever had unprotected sex or used a hypodermic needle, it is very important that you not only go for testing but also encourage your friends and family to do the same.

- Being a good neighbor involves being kind and not hurting people, but it also involves taking care of yourself in such a way that you don't spread the suffering. God may be using you to save a life—perhaps even your own.

There is an answer.
— María del Sol, singer

Responses to HIV/AIDS: Making Progress

A recent study performed by the Institute for Latino Studies at the University of Notre Dame—undertaken on behalf of Esperanza USA—revealed a lingering belief among some Hispanic church leaders that you have to be gay to get AIDS. If you've read this far into the book, you know that those particular ministers are mistaken. Thankfully, they are also part of a shrinking group.

An even more recent follow-up study, also conducted by Notre Dame's Institute for Latino Studies, found that a high percentage of Hispanic ministers had posted HIV/AIDS material in their churches. It also found that many had brought in speakers to address the topic, that parishioners reported receiving HIV information at church, and that an overwhelming majority of those same parishioners thought it was entirely appropriate for the church to get involved in giving out information about HIV/AIDS. (A copy of this study is available at www.esperanza.us.)

There are, on the other hand, some stark facts for Latinos in the United States.

- Hispanic children account for 26 percent of all new pediatric AIDS cases in the United States (NAPWA/CDC).

- Although Hispanics make up just under 14 percent of the population, they make up more than 20 percent of all new AIDS cases throughout the country.

- As we mentioned earlier, AIDS has become the second leading cause of death for Hispanic men under age fifty, and the fourth leading cause of death for Hispanic women under age fifty.

- While statistics regarding AIDS have improved in other communities, they continue to worsen in the Hispanic community.

Yes, AIDS was first identified in the gay community. Yes, the initial ravages were worst among urban Anglo men. However, a lot has happened over the last twenty years. HIV/AIDS does not follow a script. The virus does not look at your beliefs, your gender, your lifestyle, your ethnicity, or your good intentions and plans for your life.

In no way do I want the work that we do at Esperanza USA to belittle the very serious concerns about HIV among other groups—African-Americans, youth, and, as we saw in the previous chapter, whole nations across the Atlantic. But our mandate at Esperanza is to address issues affecting the Hispanic community, and to mobilize Hispanics themselves to address those issues.

There is a long-standing institution with particular organizing power in the Hispanic community. Located "on the ground" in many of the neighborhoods where HIV/AIDS has reared its head, this institution has the trust of the people, and in many cases is accessible every day around the clock, or at least on a regular basis throughout the week. This institution, for the most part, offers its services free, and it has proven staying power—no matter what kinds of problems assault it, it will not dry up and go away. It won't disappear simply because it lost a grant or its founder retired.

Of course, I am referring to the church. The Hispanic church has been called a "sleeping giant" in regard to HIV/AIDS.

The researchers at Notre Dame recently helped us ask some questions in a project called Faith-Based Response to HIV/AIDS in the U.S. Latino Community: A Needs Assessment. The point of this study, with its long academic title, was to find out three things: (1) What did pastors and leaders know about HIV/AIDS? (2) Did they think that they or their congregations had any business getting involved with it? (3) If they wanted to get involved, did they have ideas about what to do that would be helpful?

What the researchers learned was that everyone knew someone who either was HIV-positive or had died of AIDS. They learned that for ministers, not knowing what to do was more of a hindrance than not wanting to do anything. No one really believed that AIDS was not a matter for the church. All the respondents said, both to interviewers and to one another in focus groups, that they struggled more with how, where, and when to introduce information than with whether or not to try at all.

In one respect, it makes no sense that we've had to invent organizations and structures just to deal with HIV/AIDS. People with HIV/AIDS need pretty much the same things as people with any other health concerns: encouragement; health care; assistance if they are in economic need; respite for their family responsibilities when they become weakened; prayer or whatever spiritual support makes the most sense to them; clean water; safe housing; good nutrition. It is a shame that churches—as community-based organizations, which are already established contact points for people—have not been able to respond more consistently to this particular issue.

The church in general has played a positive role in the epidemic. Many church people have been doing good work, putting feet to their faith since the start. But how many parishioners have been forced to suffer in silence simply because there is still no acceptable way to even talk about HIV/AIDS in church? How many HIV infections have not been caught early, simply because people were paralyzed by fear of the truth? The very core of Christian belief is that people can change and that God readily accepts people who want to change in a positive way. The nature of HIV/AIDS is that it lies dormant for years. How can churches open their doors to people looking for new approaches to life and not expect that many will bring HIV/AIDS with them?

In a telling interview conducted by the Notre Dame researchers, one woman told of her church's progression in responding to the fact that people in the congregation were dying from this disease:

> The first stage was silence. . . . People were passing away. We went to their funerals, but there was a silence. We knew something was happening. The second stage was awareness, where I was able to bring some health care [workers] to do workshops with the leadership early on in the process; and it happened that it was a secret workshop, because they didn't trust the person who was doing it—you know, coming in and talking about AIDS, condoms, this and that. Then there was the third phase, when my pastor started saying, "You know, we have to do something about this."

I will say this: our studies and experiences show that Hispanics have some cause to feel envious of the response of the African-American and Anglo communities, including the churches, to the problem of HIV/AIDS, both in the United States and overseas. We recognize that Anglos, African-Americans, and groups in the gay community have received much more public and private funding to deal with this problem than groups based in Hispanic communities. When it comes to getting information to Hispanics, lack of public and private funding is more problematic, as we are also trying to jump the hurdles of lower academic achievement, language barriers, and less access to mainstream media and communications.

The most positive models in African-American and Anglo communities include monthly health screenings at churches, elders and leaders who are trained to give counsel and referrals, worship and prayer services at which the topic is addressed, and fund-raising for work overseas. We have found that some well-established denominational churches, including those in Hispanic communities, have attempted to respond and have begun providing education and respite ministries to their congregations and communities. Unfortunately, too many denominations and some independent councils of evangelical and Pentecostal churches continue to proceed as if they existed in a world without HIV/AIDS. Those who have wanted to act don't have the confidence to step up, or the knowledge of how to go about it.

Preliminary findings in a follow-up study of Hispanic pastors and parishioners in the Chicago area found that many had discovered ways to take initial steps: of the pastors interviewed, 47 percent said they had posted information in church about HIV/AIDS, and 38 percent had brought in a special speaker to address the topic. Among parishioners, 41 percent said they had received information about HIV/AIDS from their churches, and 79 percent believed it was right for the church to be involved with the issue in some way.

The idea that the Latino church is not engaged may no longer be true, but we remain far behind other groups. Ours is a culture that is not as open to dialogue on sexual issues; a community where a large portion of the people do not speak or understand the English language well; and a community that has had fewer resources available for those willing to do the work, to develop and distribute information, and to set up ministries like those in other American communities. There is still a wall of silence. Every human being must be educated so that we may stem the growth of this epidemic.

In the Hispanic community, people are getting sick and dying because we are losing the battleground of the mind. Not everyone is a doctor, a health professional, or an administrator of service delivery. Not everyone has HIV/AIDS, and not everyone will get it. Everyone, however, gives out information at some point in his or her life—to children or other family members, neighbors, coworkers, students, and even strangers sitting nearby on a bus. The more truth we know, the more truth we spread. The more truth we spread, the more lives will be saved.

"There are great possibilities that haven't been addressed," says Dr. Edwin Hernandez, who led the team that produced the Notre Dame report. "The church has not been mobilized, and there is great potential. There is a need for bridge builders between people affected and the church. It's critically important. These churches are precisely in the communities where the epidemic is going on."

Our study points out a truth that others have sensed for years: there is a gulf between the organizations that rose up specifically in response to AIDS, and other institutions.

For various reasons, there is often conflict between so-called AIDS activists and the many large, established social institutions that they perceived as too slow or uncaring at the start of the epidemic. The medical establishment, the pharmaceutical companies, the government, the media, and, yes, the church, have all been accused of being heartless toward dying people. Activists disrupting mass at stately St. Patrick's Cathedral a few years ago made for sensational news copy, but they did not bring about a solution, save the dying, or even enlighten befuddled worshippers who didn't see how disrupting a church service would make anybody healthier. On the other hand, many people with HIV or AIDS have slunk silently away from congregations, just as confused by the walls of silence, rejection, or, in the worst cases, condemnation.

If we want to talk about AIDS in church, we have to do it in a way that incorporates a commitment to compassion with the commitment to the values of the particular faith community. This has proved challenging in the past.

If we examine responses to HIV/AIDS around the world, we will find different definitions of success. Some international agencies consider it a success when condom sales increase in a given region; others define success by the number of "sex workers" who have enrolled in health care programs. And then there are those who consider it major progress when every man, woman, and child in a nation can hold a frank discussion about the details of HIV transmission. Documents support the fact that when clean needles are made available in areas of high intravenous drug use, the HIV infection rate goes down.

Perhaps the church that is aware, active, and willing to help can develop its own measure of success in HIV/AIDS involvement by considering the following. How many HIV-positive people have been successfully integrated into the full life of the community? Have they visited services? Have they been invited to small group or cell meetings? Have they made friends? Have their children been successfully welcomed into kids' programs and made friends? Do people in the congregation operate with an awareness of HIV/AIDS? Are families that have been directly affected by HIV as free to share this problem with church staff members, in prayer meetings, or in support groups as they might be with any other problem? Are there sermons to relieve the families' pain? Is there counseling available for the family of an HIV or AIDS patient?

Pain, guilt, fear, and spiritual comfort and counseling on issues such as an afterlife are all part of what the church can do. Add to this physical items such as food, shelter, and clothing—things that are sometimes greatly needed. Finally, too many people with HIV/AIDS are abandoned by their family, friends, and coworkers. What greater service is there than to just be a friend, to be the only community to extend a handshake or hug in the name of God to a person who has been abandoned by all but God?

These are just suggestions. As we are learning in our ongoing research, when people think differently, they act differently. And when people are active, they are creative. What a difference this could make!

*   *   *

Keeping informed on health issues in this day and age can seem very complicated. With so much being published on the Internet and in the many other kinds of media available, you may ask yourself how you can judge what is good information, what is erroneous, and what is just plain propaganda.

First of all, let me applaud you for having read this book. It shows that your heart is in the right place. Now, if you would like your head to keep up with your heart, please take advantage of the advice in the following pages about where to seek further information. Among the topics addressed are:

- *Caring for your own health.*

- *Being a support to a loved one.*

- *Becoming active in your community.*

- *Making a difference in the epidemic globally.*

Most important, whether you or someone you know has HIV/AIDS, or even if you're one among the many people who simply want to educate themselves about this epidemic, realize this:

There is an answer.
— Julissa, singer

PART 4

False Comfort

"Delia, Hector is really upset over this whole thing. I'm with you, girl, but I have to live with him. He is adamant. No one from my house is allowed anywhere near your family. Not just Marc; you and the kids, too. I told him that he is a hardheaded idiot, but he is putting me through hell over this. Mama is really mad at both of us, and it looks like now I'll have to cook for myself this Thanksgiving. So, I am going to put something extra in Hector's *gandules* that he will not like."

Delia could hardly believe what Sandra was telling her over the phone. She had always been so close to Marc's aunt, and now their relationship was on the brink of falling apart. Worse, she wasn't even sure who she should be maddest at: Hector, for keeping his family away; Sandra, for letting him do so; or Marc, for contracting HIV and causing this entire mess.

Sandra's voice cut into her thoughts. "Delia? I'm sorry, you know? You believe me, right, honey?"

"Okay, Sandra," she answered, trying to hide her disappointment. "So, what else is happening with you?"

"Well, we're good. Hector just got a raise, and you heard that my Susie's expecting, right? We know she's young, but she married a good guy. He had good training in the military and as long as he stays on reserve status, they'll be happy. We just hope he doesn't get called up or sent overseas, you know?"

"Yes, that would be rough."

A brief, uncomfortable silence suddenly fell between them. Finally Sandra asked, "So, are you going to be okay?"

"Sandra, one day at a time, you know." Delia couldn't hold back any longer; she had to ask. "Tell me something: does the whole family know already?"

"Yes, everybody knows. You know how this family is. One stubs his toe and they *all* say 'Ouch.' "

"What are they saying? About Marc?"

"Oh, you know me, I don't listen to gossip." It was clear in Sandra's voice that she didn't want to be put on the spot. "I don't want to be around them. They were all at Mama's the other day, but I wasn't there."

"Sandra, listen to me. We haven't told the kids everything yet. We are giving information to them piece by piece. I don't want anybody spilling everything to them. We're over the initial shock now. Marc is setting up appointments with a minister and the clinic, and I've been to the doctor, so we have a shot at a pretty normal life for a while. I want the kids to have that. This family can at least help me with that."

"Did Mama—Grandma—call you?" Sandra asked. Everybody—even Sandra, sometimes—referred to her mother as "Grandma," because she was clearly the matriarch of the family.

"She did, but just to invite us over. She doesn't like talking on the phone, you know, so I really don't know what she's thinking. She did send over a gallon of soup."

"Well, like I said, she's really mad at Hector. And me, because she says I should stand up to him. But I have my problems too, you know, honey? I've got to look out for what's going on around here. My Susie's baby is coming, you know?"

Delia didn't respond. What could she say?

"Hey, let me know if I can do anything for you, okay? I'd better go. Hector's going to be home soon. Bye, honey, okay?"

"Bye, Sandra."

Delia hung up the phone and started to cry.

A Pastoral Perspective

Marc walked into the church. It had been some time since he had last been there—several years, in fact; not since his oldest child's dedication—but the smell of flowers was the same. He wasn't sure where the pastor's office was until a custodian pointed down the stairs. His footsteps sounded a bit loud as he descended. The door marked "Clergy" creaked as he opened it. Inside sat Pastor Estrada, who didn't look older than Marc remembered him, though it was clear that the pastor would no longer play basketball.

Hey, that's a good place to start the conversation, Marc thought. *Basketball, and then move it to—*

"Marcus!" the pastor shouted. "God bless you, my son. I am so happy to see you! It has been a while. And to what miracle do I owe this visit?" he asked, laughing. "Are you having another child? I would love to hear that! *Y tú mama . . .* Well, let me let you do the talking, Marcus."

"Well, ahh . . ." Marc hesitated, trying to think of something to say. "Ma is fine, and so is Abuela. I am sorry that I haven't been around, Pastor, but . . . well, you know how it is."

Marc regretted coming, but now it was too late. He wasn't sure what to do or how to say it.

Pastor Estrada could tell there was a more serious matter at hand. "Marcus, why don't we pray together?"

I don't know what to say, Marc thought as the pastor started praying. *I agreed with Delia to do this, and I know Pastor Estrada is cool and wouldn't be nasty or look down his nose or scold me, but I need to figure out how to—*

". . . Amen!" said the pastor, further embarrassing Marc. *I didn't hear much of the prayer.*

Desperate to avoid the unavoidable, Marc asked, "Uh, Pastor, do you still play ball?"

"Yes, Marcus, but never mind that. Your spirit tells me something is up. There is nothing you can say that will change God's love for you, or my commitment to serve you and your family."

"Really." Resigned, Marc blurted out, almost casually, "Well, Pastor, how about I've got HIV, my time on this planet is limited, and I'm not sure about God right now, though I think I'd better get my act together real soon? You know—life . . . death . . . my kids . . . my wife . . ."

"Marcus, do you have AIDS or HIV?"

His comment took Marc completely by surprise. *Wow, a good question from the pastor,* he thought, then replied, "HIV. And I don't want the world to know."

Pastor Estrada reached across the desk and grabbed Marc's

hand. "Let's pray together, Marcus. Let's hold hands and ask God for relief . . . relief from your future burdens, relief for your family, relief from your sin . . . relief from the burden of your ill health . . ."

The two men prayed, then sat in silence for a long time. Finally, out of nowhere, the pastor noted, "You know, Marcus, you must use a condom for the rest of your life. With Delia or with another, if you decide to sin with another."

The pastor spoke so matter-of-factly that it took Marc a second to become embarrassed; the words had been cold, yet so true. *I will be reminded of this every time I hold my wife*, he told himself. *If I could go back in time . . .*

Then words came out of his mouth, things he had never told even Delia. Marc let go of so much that the tears streaming from his eyes felt as if they were cleansing him. He had been reminded that God so loved the world that He gave His only begotten son so that who believed in Him would not perish. *I am not alone*, he realized. *God puts a value on me. I am a child of God, and I have work to do. I have a mission and a vocation. I have a role to play as a husband and father, neighbor and friend.* Pastor Estrada had confirmed God's presence in Marc's life, and it brought about a great peace.

The pastor then mentioned the small group of HIV/AIDS folks he had Bible study with. Marc thought it was pretty cool for a pastor to do that, but said that he wasn't yet ready for that. He made an appointment to come back in a few weeks. As he rose to leave, the pastor also got up, came around the desk, and gave him a great big hug.

"I love you, Marcus," he said, "and God does too. And we love your family—Delia and the kids are not alone. Until you are ready, your condition is our secret."

Strange, Marc noticed, *no one has ever held me like this. Not even family members, except Delia.*

His steps up the stairs felt so light, as if a thousand pounds had been taken off his neck and chest. *God does love me*, he kept telling himself. *God is present in my life, even under these circumstances. God will not abandon me. He will be with me every step of the way.*

"Hey, Marcus!" the pastor hollered as he reached the top step. "I still want to see you in church on Sunday. My sermons aren't *that* bad."

Marc couldn't help laughing out loud. "I hear you, Pastor! Maybe I'll come on Sunday."

* * *

What would Jesus do in the age of HIV/AIDS?

Some say the church should stick to preaching against sin and not venture into dealing with "worldly matters." Others say the church is so clueless that it couldn't be of any help, anyway.

The fact is that from the beginning of the epidemic, 40 percent of the agencies caring for those with HIV/AIDS around the world have been faith-based organizations.

It's not always easy to know how to respond. There are serious questions. At least now we're talking and starting to find some answers.

What would Jesus do in the age of HIV/AIDS? The same things He did when He was here. Be with people. Tell the truth. Spread healing.

I'm up for that. How about you?

There is an answer.
— *The Reverend Luis Cortés Jr.*

PART 5

More Bad News

Delia was on the phone to Sandra as soon as she heard. "We are here for you," was all she wanted to say. She knew she might get a double dose of rejection hurled back at her, but she would not risk leaving anybody alone with this thing. At least people had to believe she could understand. But Sandra was angry.

"This is *your* fault," she told Delia, almost spitting through her sobs at the other end of the receiver. "If you guys had kept this to yourselves, the rest of us would never be going through this now. We were fine, and now we have to deal with this."

The other day, Grandma had arranged HIV tests for the entire family. Hector had not wanted to do it, but Sandra, who was tired of being harangued by her mother and the rest of the family, had insisted. "What's the big deal, anyway?" she had told him. "Neither of us has it."

However, Hector and Sandra had both tested positive. Follow-up testing had shown that Hector's white blood cell count was very low.

"I'm so mad," Sandra snarled at the other end of the phone. "I wish I was over there just so I could spit in your face. I hope you get it, too, Delia. You are so . . ." She couldn't finish the tirade because she had started sobbing.

"Delia . . . I'm sorry," Sandra said, regaining her composure somewhat. "I know it's not your fault. I just don't understand. Why should I have HIV? Why? And Hector . . . he's so advanced. He's got it bad and it could break out into something serious any minute. They're not even sure the medicines will work. As it is, we're living paycheck to paycheck. We're about to be grandparents. I just don't know how we're going to do this."

"Sandra," Delia said softly, "I just want you to know I am here to talk, to help you, to walk along with you. At least you won't be afraid of us anymore. I want to be your friend. And besides, we're family. We have learned so much."

Marc came up behind his wife and wrapped an arm around her shoulders. "Who are you talking to?" he whispered.

"It's Sandra."

"Give me the phone." Delia handed him the receiver. "Hey, little *tia*. How's it going?"

"Marc, Marc . . ." she answered her nephew. "I am so sorry, Marcus. I love you, little boy. Can you forgive me?"

"Sandi, calm down. You know I'm a guy and crying makes me nervous. Of course I forgive you. And you'll stay forgiven if you do one thing for me."

"What's that, Marcus?"

"Keep talking to me and let us help you guys in whatever way we can. Tell Hector I am coming to see him this weekend, whether he likes it or not."

Hector told Marc to meet him at the diner near the construction site around lunchtime. Hector didn't want to miss dinner at home. He liked to keep things as routine as possible—at home, at work, everywhere. Breaking routine started conversation, which sooner or later ended up involving questions. Hector didn't like conversation, and he certainly didn't like questions. But his nephew wasn't going to leave him alone about this, so he agreed to meet for lunch; this way, there was limited time, and there were no women around to get involved in their talk.

Hector walked into the small entry foyer of the busy diner exactly on time. Marc came in a couple of minutes past one.

"Hey, *tio*, man. *¿Qué tal?*" Marc said as he slapped his uncle on the back.

"Great, Marc. Listen, I've got to start back in half an hour, okay?"

"No sweat, bro. I just want to have lunch with you, you know?"

"Let's get a table, then."

The waitress approached their little booth in the corner almost as soon as they sat down. She and the lunchtime crowd were all in a hurry. Though perhaps, Marc thought, not as much as his uncle seemed to be.

"Well, I already know what I want," Marc said. "Could you bring me a spinach salad and some water—but not in a glass. Bottled, please. Plus, I want a huge fruit salad"—he held his cupped hands out to mime a large-sized bowl—"like this, you know? But after, okay? You can do that?" He smiled at the waitress.

"Yeah, sure," the waitress said as she scribbled on her notepad. "And you?" She looked at Hector, her pen poised and ready to write.

"Yeah, bring me that, too," he said, flat and emotionless.

The waitress left and the two men sat without speaking for a few minutes. Marc drummed his fingers on the table. Hector sat stone-faced, waiting for Marc to say something; it was Marc who had insisted that they meet, so it was up to him to start talking. But Marc just sat, drummed his fingers again, smiled pleasantly, and looked around the diner.

Their order came quickly. The waitress set salad and water down in front of each of them. Hector stared at Marc as he picked up his fork and started eating.

"Well, you seem happy," Hector said. It was an accusation.

"Hey, you know what? Since I've been following all this advice the nutritionist gave me, I've been feeling pretty good—"

"You jerk," Hector whispered loudly, banging his fork down on the table. "You're sick. Don't play around with me, man. You're sick. I'm sick. What the hell is wrong with you?"

"I'm HIV-positive," Marc said.

"Shhh! You want someone to hear you?"

"Hector, man, it's not a crime. I'm no danger to anyone. It doesn't matter who hears."

"Well, shut up and eat."

They were quiet again for a few minutes. Finally, Marc said, "Hector, I didn't come here to eat, you know."

"Well, what do you want?"

"I want you to see that you have some life left in you, that you can live and appreciate it. I came to ask you if you've been to the doctor—a *good* doctor."

"I went to the clinic," Hector said, still looking around to see if anyone else was listening. "I shouldn't have, but I didn't want to make any more of a scene in the family. Now they pronounce this death sentence over me. What the hell else do you want me to do?"

"Come see my guy. He knows a lot more about this than most doctors."

"What is there to know? I'm going to *die*. Maybe he can tell me how soon, or maybe he can ask a lot of questions about my past or put me on some stupid diet. I'm a man, Marc. I want to die like a man. Do my work, eat my food, sleep in my bed, and then die like a man. I deserve what's happening to me. I brought it on myself a long time ago. Sandi doesn't ask me, and I haven't told her. But we're men. When she was pregnant with Susie, I started going to prostitutes, okay? Maybe it happened when I did a little drugs, but I was never a junkie. Who knew anything about this? I'm a man and this is what happened. I just . . . I feel so bad about Sandi . . ."

He didn't finish his sentence. He had already said a lot more than he had intended to. He had barely touched his food. He asked the waitress for some coffee.

"Hector," Marc assured him, "there's no such thing as somebody who deserves to get HIV. I don't deserve it. You don't, and my *tia* Sandi sure doesn't deserve it."

"Don't mention her . . ."

"Hector, she is part of this story. This is one thing you are not the boss over. If you want to live in a prison of pride and pretending, that's up to you. But you can't keep Sandi in there with you. So you're not proud of your past. Me neither. There's time to get that straight, and there's every reason to live as healthy as you can for as long as you can. You're not proud of your past right now. So start making a past you *can* be proud of. Do the right thing by yourself, your wife, your family. God."

"Oh, now you're going to mention God? *You?*"

"Well, I've been talking to a minister, you know? To straighten myself out. Me and Delia, we are getting better together, even if I still don't know what's going to happen to me. Who knows how many years I have left, but I want them to count for something. I'm a man too, Hector. I want to do my work, eat the right food, talk to my wife and kids every night about the real things in life. And I want people to be at peace at my funeral, not all torn up and not knowing what to say."

Hector stared at Marc for a minute, trying to decide whether or not to get any further into the conversation.

Finally, all he said was, "It's late. I've got to go."

*   *   *

What I do matters.

I can protect myself, my family, my community, and my country from a threat worse than terrorism.

I will not take it lightly when a friend or relative belittles his spouse or partner.

I will not laugh it off when a friend is so drunk or so high that he puts at risk his own life and the lives of those who are close to him.

I refuse to be amused when "the guys" brag about risky sexual adventures.

I will do my part to stop the cycle of HIV/AIDS infection: taking a test, finding treatment, helping friends to do the same. It's all good.

I want my sisters to live and be well.

I want all our children to live with hope and a future.

I want my brothers to be strong, healthy men who bring good— not disease and hopelessness—to our communities.

I'm an answer.
—*Marcos Witt, singer*

Becoming Part of the Solution

Fighting HIV/AIDS doesn't always mean taking a test or dispensing medicine. Sometimes it means helping a family fix their home or pay the rent. It can mean delivering clean water to places where the supply has been destroyed or contaminated. It can even mean being quiet and listening before giving advice or offering a prayer.

Nancy Rivera, founder and director of Sembrando Flores in Florida, is known for her expertise in housing issues. In fact, she has so much credibility with her county's housing authority it has given her office space. She, her staff, and volunteers—both local residents and a steady stream of out-of-state visitors—have renovated a number of homes in the Miami-Dade area they serve. Recently, they were instrumental in delivering relief to inner-city and hard-to-reach rural communities whose water supplies, power sources, and food deliveries were cut off by hurricane Katrina. Over the years, Sembrando has also provided thousands of simple HIV tests to people who would otherwise probably never have requested them.

Ms. Rivera first showed up in Florida in 1992, as a volunteer setting up housing for the elderly and the poor in the aftermath of hurricane Andrew. Eventually, the housing authority sent her out into the community, to see if the programs and services it was providing were actually doing the job.

"I dressed like the people," she recalls, "visited them at home and work, and found out that many issues were not being addressed. I met many, many families living with HIV, and dying without ever having medical intervention or counseling. I saw HIV in the children and family sector. Many women were losing their children because of neglect, but it was because they were sick. That's when I became an advocate on HIV/AIDS and family violence.

"People come to us for many things," Ms. Rivera adds. "It's not always about the money." But, she points out, people are not going to tell their entire life story to someone they have just met. "Once you start the dialogue, the other things come out."

Her agency is prepared to provide testing and counseling—an RN (resident nurse), a professional counselor, and a teacher are on the staff. But HIV/AIDS is not on the sign on the front door. "Our first year, we gave out cards that said HIV/AIDS Latino Ministries," she explains. "People ran away."

She continues, "At first, all I wanted to do was work with Latinos who were infected, but God had a bigger plan." That plan entailed Ms. Rivera taking her background in housing and community advocacy, and her deep concern that serious hidden needs were still going unaddressed, and entwining them into the holistic outreach known as Sembrando Flores. "If the need is feeding, we feed. If it's clothing, we clothe. If it's a distressed building, we go get paint and we fix it."

Nancy Rivera and Sembrando Flores have also built relationships beyond the Hispanic community. They have gotten to know the entire "salad of ethnicities" in the region they serve, which includes Haitian and African-American people, as well as individuals from all walks of life, from agricultural workers to middle-class professionals. "What I tell the team is that we're here to serve whoever walks in that door," she says, realizing that to address the issue of HIV/AIDS at the community level "without being threatening . . . It's a long, long process."

Paying rent, painting homes, and delivering food and water are how Nancy Rivera often works to combat HIV/AIDS.

Nils Arne Kastberg runs the Latin American division of

UNICEF. UNICEF, of course, is a huge global subdivision of the even larger global agency known as the United Nations. The UN has an entire division called UNAIDS, devoted to AIDS information and action.

Kastberg, who was raised in South America, has as his mission the well-being of children. Since the turn of the millennium, he notes, there is very little of UNICEF's work that has not been affected by HIV/AIDS. Beyond the staggering fact that there are 750,000 AIDS orphans in Latin America, there is the issue of nutrition for newborns. Everyone knows that the healthiest food for a newborn is mother's milk, provided the mother has been well cared for. When a mother is HIV-positive—as are an increasing number of women of childbearing age in Latin America and the Caribbean—the question of counseling the mother to nurse her baby or use a supplement arises. Breast milk does carry HIV. Formula, on the other hand, is a practical and healthy option only where good water is available.

Sometimes Nils Arne Kastberg fights AIDS by strategizing with heads of state to coordinate care and intervention for women and children, and to reduce the number of young teenage mothers by means of various educational and family support projects. Sometimes, however, like Nancy Rivera, Nils Arne Kastberg fights AIDS simply by delivering water.

Dr. Ramón Gadea, the physician who used to run Esperanza's health clinic in North Philadelphia, has known about AIDS since before he was a doctor. When he was a child, his aunt died, unattended, in a hospital emergency room in Puerto Rico, because the staff members on duty were afraid to touch her. Not long ago, he came face-to-face with what the epidemic has been doing to the Dominican Republic. Rather than wait to strategize at the national level, Dr. Gadea set up and personally funds a small clinic in San Pedro de Macorís, giving proceeds from his training on behalf of pharmaceutical companies. He hopes the clinic and the model established there will be replicated, either within his own organization—Access Caribe—or outside it. But for now, he is doing all he can to make this one health station a success.

Sometimes people fight AIDS by taking care of the sick.

There comes a time when assisting people with AIDS means giving comfort to the dying. Reverend Rosa Caraballo was a pastor's wife in the Bronx when she first met a person with AIDS. She had been brought up in a churchgoing military family. In the early 1980s, members of her congregation were the first to come to her for help in dealing with the multiple issues presented by the presence of HIV/AIDS in the family.

People who know her work in later years—as a hospital chaplain and director of an outreach for Hispanic women whose families have been affected by HIV/AIDS—are generally astounded by the amount of on-the-job training she went through in the early days. She studied, collected information, and got to know people in the community so that she could be better prepared to help those who were counting on her. What was set in motion then has not stopped to this day; she has maintained herself as an advocate of, spokesperson for, and friend to families dealing with AIDS.

Reverend Rosa Caraballo and several other women she has worked with are now telling their stories in *Covenant of Hope: A Woman's Healing Journey in the AIDS Epidemic*. This bilingual book, full of personal stories and practical information, was recently published, I am proud to say, under a grant from Esperanza USA. I am even prouder to know a woman such as Rosa Caraballo, who years ago refused to pass the buck. Instead, she took on a challenge, and she has since then quietly comforted and assisted hundreds of families. You can get more information about this book at www.esperanza.us.

Sometimes you fight AIDS by turning yourself into a knowledgeable counselor and friend.

What Can I Personally Do?

Anytime you want to accomplish a goal, you have to break it into steps. If you were enrolling in school, you wouldn't try to learn everything you need to know all at once. Let's imagine that becoming aware, healthy, and in some way involved in a world with HIV/AIDS is like going to school. I have to start with the basics— "HIV/AIDS 101." Next, I decide how much further I want to go in my education, with no feeling of shame if I stop when I have reached my capacity for the moment. Of course, there is also no shame in offering advanced courses, or in choosing to pursue them. Remember, any work you do may at some point bring you into contact with a need related to HIV/AIDS. The more prepared you are, the more effective you will be in responding.

Course titles for students at level one could include these:

- "Educating Myself." This course will cover the following topics—What is AIDS? When did it originate and start to spread? How is it transmitted today? A class project I would strongly suggest would be to visit the Esperanza USA website, where you can find fact sheets on HIV/AIDS. Get started at www.esperanza.us and go to Programs\Pacto de Esperanza.

- "Taking Care of Myself." How do I take care not to contract HIV? How do I take care not to transmit it?

For students at level two:

- "Developing Awareness and Etiquette." Being frank and informed on the issue of HIV/AIDS does not mean being insensitive or rude. Learn how to share the facts without running roughshod over people. Learn how to become a resource others can trust.

- "Educating and Taking Care of My Family." Where are HIV tests offered in my area? Who should be tested? What are some likely reactions to learning of a positive test result? What are helpful responses?

On completing level two, I have become a person friends and family can go to for basic information when a question comes up.

At this point, students may want to consider signing the Covenant of Hope/Pacto de Esperanza that thousands nationwide have signed, demonstrating their commitment to fighting the HIV/AIDS attack on the Hispanic community. This is available at our website, www.esperanza.us.

For students at level three:

- "Becoming Aware of Community Efforts." This course educates students about meal delivery services, buddy programs, and community educator programs, as well as about becoming a support group facilitator or hospital volunteer. Course requirements will involve practical experience; students will spend at least ten hours in service opportunities.

For students at level four:

- "Becoming Aware of and Involved in International

Efforts." This course instructs students about mission organizations, international agencies, and finding ways to provide the funding and expertise—short-term and long-term—needed in these areas.

Every level completed is valuable in and of itself. If everybody does something, there is no telling how fast we might be able to reverse the spread of suffering.

I have chosen to offer one more class in my imaginary school—an advanced elective course for men only. I would love to see a similar course offered for women, but I am not qualified to teach it. I will leave it to other authorities to design and implement such a course. Women are welcome to audit my class, as are men who are not yet sure whether they want to get this advanced in their commitment to working to stop the spread of HIV/AIDS.

For (Brave) Men Only

Imagine that you're walking down the street in your own neighborhood. Your wife is with you. You are laughing in a way you haven't done in a while as you take a walk to the little restaurant a few blocks away. It's just getting dark as you cross the street into the more commercial section where there are older, taller buildings. You step up to the curb and start to cross the concrete slabs that make up the sidewalk.

Suddenly, from between the first two buildings in the row, a guy jumps out and grabs your wife. In a flash, you know you've seen this creep hanging around near the gas station or the bar up the block. Your blood starts boiling. Before you've even had time to think, you are all over this guy, pounding on him with strength you didn't even know you had. He's on the ground, you're pounding his face with your fist, hoping you draw blood. He flips you over, and now you're lying on your back on the sidewalk. You come out of your rage just long enough to realize he might kill you before you kill him. Your nose is bleeding and your head hurts. He's sitting on top of you. You're pushing this guy until every muscle you have is tensed and flexed. He is like a rock and won't budge. You don't give up, though. You'll find the strength or you'll die trying because this is your woman, your family, your life.

Gentlemen, we need to talk. The numbers are in. HIV/AIDS is stalking Hispanic women and children.

How do children get HIV/AIDS? Young children generally become HIV-positive in only one way: from an HIV-positive mother during pregnancy or childbirth. Exceptions to this are exceedingly rare, and grave—either the child has been sexually abused in some way, or the child has come into contact with contaminated blood.

Medication is available to significantly lower the risk of transmission during birth, though at least two things stop women from taking advantage of this: either they do not have the money for proper medical care for themselves, or they don't know they are infected. Rules governing HIV testing in the United States vary from state to state. In some states, all prisoners are automatically tested. In some hospitals, patients who are admitted are tested. But most practices still depend heavily on a person's deciding to ask for or submit to testing. For people to take an HIV test, they usually need to have some reason to think that they might be infected.

Hispanic children get HIV from their mothers. How do Hispanic women get HIV? By and large, the numbers show that Hispanic women get HIV from men, not from needles or transfusions.

I am not trying to be paternalistic, and I don't want to come off as chauvinistic. (I'm not.) I only want to be realistic. There are several ways that HIV is transmitted, but the top three remain: male homosexual intercourse, sharing infected needles, and male-female sexual contact.

The government and the church can each do their part, and the medical establishment can do what it does best. But there is a part that only we, the men in our community, can play.

We see a lot of numbers in the work we do at Esperanza USA, but the stories we hear have had an even greater impact on me. Any story of someone who becomes sick because of HIV is sad, but I see an extra tragedy in the accounts we hear, far too often, in which a woman becomes infected because the man she lives with and trusts brings the infection from outside the house into the home, and into her body.

If this happened once and we knew about it, that would be enough cause for this woman's brothers to rise up and take action. But this scenario is repeated all too often in the United States and Latin America. Some men may do this without realizing they themselves carry HIV. Too many others are fully aware of their own condition, and yet they are unwilling to let their partners know.

There are laws in the United States that carry penalties for knowingly spreading HIV. But we don't hear very many cases in which family members have brought charges against people they love for bringing illness into their lives. Yes, we are also aware that women have carelessly infected sexual partners without warning them of the risks. But the numbers, at the moment, skew in the direction of male-to-female infection.

If you carry the HIV virus or have AIDS, you must have the moral conscience to protect your sexual partner. You must not

only educate yourself about the disease but also educate and protect others.

Again, thousands of people have already signed the Covenant
of Hope that we promote on our website and at regional meetings on HIV/AIDS. Please consider joining the ranks of those who
want to be part of the solution, not part of the problem. Go to
www.esperanza.us and sign the Covenant of Hope/Pacto de Esperanza.

PART 6

The Final Hours

The staff in the hospital's AIDS unit had a special meeting about the family. The patient in 412B was very sick, and very cranky. Yet he had so many visitors that the staff had to plan for them in the daily routines. Somebody showed up every time visiting was allowed. The patient's mother-in-law and wife were there most often, but to make sure he never went without visitors, the whole family took turns. So the staff was often confronted with somebody new who had to be trained in the precautions necessary for the good of both the patient and the visitor.

This was actually becoming such a problem that the staff started thinking about restricting visits to members of the immediate family only. They weren't sure exactly how to bring it up.

This situation usually didn't happen, and nobody knew whether or not to make a real issue of it. The staff could hear that the patient wasn't always very nice to those who came to see him, but they could also see that he usually ate and slept a little better after members of the family had visited. They kept coming and taking turns. It was an unusual phenomenon in the AIDS unit: a patient with too many visitors.

One day, the doctor had a particularly heavy report for the patient's wife. She left the unit crying and headed straight to the only place she knew she'd be safe enough to let go and deal with things: her mother's kitchen.

"Mama, he was unconscious today." Sandra was shaking a little as she clutched a cup of tea, trying to warm up and steady her nerves. "He couldn't talk to me. He doesn't even look like himself. He is so little, so weak." She put the teacup aside and laid her head down on her mother's kitchen table.

"Oh, Sandra. Oh, child." Grandma said this over and over as she stroked her daughter's hair. Then she whispered something to herself—that was how she generally prayed unless someone asked her to pray out loud—before speaking again. "It is difficult for you. Honey, you know everyone has done everything possible. Even Hector cooperated once he understood the seriousness of it. Now we have to wait. And we must take care of you, too. I want you to go lie down before Marc and Delia come. Later we will come and ask you to eat something. Okay, honey?"

"Mama, I can't sleep . . ."

"I didn't say sleep. I said lie down. Go on, try."

Sandra hadn't gotten up yet when Marc and Delia came in the back way. They opened and closed the door quietly and slipped into two of the chairs at Grandma's table. Marc stayed bundled in his scarf, hat, and jacket for a while after sitting down. Lately, the cold had been getting to him a little more than usual. Sandra stayed where she was, resting her head on her arms.

"You're not alone, *mi amor*," Grandma said. "We are here."

The family had always dressed well for funerals. Their abuelo had been a workingman, but he wore a suit and tie for anything important—a wedding, a baptism, and especially a funeral. Always a suit and tie for Abuelo, right up until his own funeral, which had been many years ago. Abuela had taken care of the dark wool suit she had worn then. She made small, skillful alterations to it whenever she had needed to wear it. Each time she put it away, she took care to keep it brushed, cleaned, and hung properly.

When she took it out this time, it was for her youngest son-in-law, Hector. "This will be the first time I do this for one of my children," she said, closing her eyes and leaning against the frame of the closet door before taking the hanger completely off the rod. Delia, who had come over to help her get ready, took the heavy garment bag from her and laid it out on the bed. She unzipped the bag and took out the suit.

"Still beautiful, Abuela," she said, looking at Grandma's peaceful eyes and silver hair, arranged in perfect order.

"Thank God," she said quietly. "Let's get dressed."

A short while later, Marc picked them up for the drive to the funeral home, where he and the family would start many hours of greeting visitors. Hector's parents were both deceased; Abuela had been his only mother since his own children were small. He had a brother and sister with whom he was still in contact, and the family would probably need to offer them a lot of support. Marc's uncle, who never liked talking to begin with, had had the hardest time telling them. Once they knew, they had worked pretty hard at overcoming their strained relationship, to try to be there for him.

Grandma entered the funeral home and saw that Sandra was already there, talking to her sister, Lucy. Sandra's eyes were red and puffy, but she too had taken care with her clothes.

"Oh, Mama," she said, taking the hug her mother offered her. "Why is he leaving me now that I finally love him?"

"Abuela." It was Sandra's daughter, Susie, stepping into the hall from the little office where she had been going over last-minute arrangements with the funeral director. She walked over and kissed her grandmother. Her husband, in dress uniform, stepped out of the office, toting an infant carrier. Inside the little seat, with mounds of new blankets spilling out over the sides, lay their baby, Hector and Sandra's first grandchild.

"Abuela, he got to see the baby," Susie said, tears forming in her eyes. "I never saw him so happy."

"You did well, *mija*. You did very well. Even if he didn't say it, you know he was proud that you named your son Hector."

Grandma then looked around at the rest of her family. "Susie has honored her father's memory. Let's all do the same. Remember, we will have our time to cry at the house tomorrow. We will cry and talk tomorrow *en casa*, okay?"

The director positioned the family around the coffin and down the sides of the darkened room. Before taking their places, they stepped up to the coffin and said good-bye. They closed the heavy wooden lid before visitors came; the gaunt, pale figure, his dress clothes hanging on mere bones, was not the Hector anyone recognized. He would not have wanted anyone outside the family seeing him like that.

It was necessary to have the accordion room divider open so that there would be a double room for receiving visitors; even so, the crowd stretched from front to back along both sides of the room. The children were surprisingly quiet as they played in the back of the room. Lucy and Delia took turns sitting with them so they wouldn't get out of hand.

Everyone had been instructed to be very careful about what was said around Marc and Delia's children. They were old enough to understand a lot. By now, they knew their dad was seriously ill as well, even though he made efforts to play with them and stay as healthy as possible. At some point, they were bound to experience everything happening around them this evening in a heightened way.

The doors opened and visitors began to come, as did the usual dialogue heard at funerals. "Thank you for coming." "Yes, he was very sweet and peaceful near the end." "I know Sandi appreciates the support from the guys at work." "Thank you." "Yes, God bless you, too." "It is a hard way to go, but he had a lot of time to say his good-byes and put things in order."

Every so often, people would come through the receiving line and tell family members they were friends of Grandma's. These people, of both genders and all ages, would each say they were praying for the family, and they trusted that Hector was now completely healed and at peace.

Grandma stayed on her feet almost the entire time. Every so often, she'd tell Sandra to sit in the center seat in the front row. Grandma's pastor—who had recently become Sandra and Hector's—sat in the front row as well, sometimes talking to the young widow, at other times quietly observing the rest of the family. At the conclusion of visiting hours, he got up in front of everyone and offered a short prayer.

"Thank you, God, for having been here with us all along," he said. "We ask that you stay with us all through this long night.

We pray that your peace—the deepest peace you offer, the one we can't ever completely understand—settles over each of us tonight. Walk with us as we walk out in this last remembrance of Hector, who is past his suffering and already with you. May we respect our brother and honor you in all we say and do. Amen."

The funeral director stepped forward to dismiss everyone as diplomatically as possible, and provide instructions about where and when services would be the next morning.

Marc was one of the lead pallbearers. He had insisted, and nobody would argue with him. Everyone had to admit, anyway, that lately he had been having more good days than bad. Today, he seemed to be throwing every ounce of his strength into performing this last service for Hector.

The pallbearers set the coffin down and joined their wives and loved ones in the pews of Grandma's little church. The musicians of the church had arranged for some soft keyboard playing as the coffin was brought in, and Sandra was escorted to her seat at the front, next to Abuela.

The senior pastor—a man of about seventy—began the service with a prayer. Then, a soloist sang. Hector had not been the type to have a favorite song, so he had probably told Sandra to choose something she liked. Sandra, however, was having a hard time focusing and making decisions, so she had ultimately left details like music and flowers to Susie.

Mi anhelo, mi deseo, siempre has sido tú.

It was time for the eulogy, the final word. The senior pastor, the one who had prayed in the funeral home the night before, remained seated. His son, wearing a dark suit jacket over a black collarless shirt, stood up and approached the clear Lucite pulpit. After he had quietly greeted the congregation—family members, a few of Sandra's friends, and a surprising number of people from the church—his somewhat serious manner became a little less formal.

"I asked my dad if I could say a few words here today," he said. "Even though you don't know me well, I have gotten to know you—Hector, Sandra, Abuela, and the family—over the last few months. I weep with you on the loss of your husband, father, brother, uncle, cousin, and son-in-law. You are already missing him. You have wrestled with some difficult issues: Hector's physical pain and suffering, as well as your own emotions as you have had to deal openly with things that were hidden for a long time. You are tired from all the thinking and talking that has been required of you, from confronting the uncertain as well as the certain. No amount of silver and gold will repair and restore what this has cost you. As far as I know, your strength will be renewed only as you lean toward the Lord.

"I don't know where each and every one of you stands with God today. But I asked my dad if I could speak because I really wanted to communicate this to you. Whether you know it or not, whether it matters to you or not, the way you have cared for Hector and interacted as a family has been exactly the picture God paints of how His people are designed to interact. He says, 'As the body is one and has many members, so also is Christ. . . . And if one member suffers, all the members suffer with it; or if one member is honored, all the members rejoice with it.' I have been taught this all my life, but I don't know if I have ever seen it demonstrated the way I have seen it over these past several months. I believe God will honor the care you have given, the love you have shown, the selflessness that has been evident. I know you have had days when you have said things out of anger or thought things of which you are ashamed. Know that God is ready to forgive it all, as ready as He is to glorify Himself and place you in honor as you have honored Him and His ways—again, whether you know it or not.

"Church family," he concluded, "I want to include you in this as well: your care and attention to Señora San Rafael, to her daughter and son-in-law, and to the rest of her family has made me proud not only to be a pastor in this church, but just to be a part of this church at all. They were relatively new among us. They came with a serious need. And they found a place where they could speak about that need—HIV/AIDS in their family—and be received and welcomed and encouraged and helped. I am proud to know all of you, and I am proud to be one of you."

Everyone was quiet. The musicians began to play again; it was the song that had been sung earlier. The soloist quietly invited any who knew it to join him, and most of the church parishioners started singing. No one in the family was quite up to it but, as many of them told each other later, they liked being surrounded by the music at that moment.

De mañana te buscaré y sé que te hallaré.

At a signal from the pastor, Marc and the other pallbearers stood and took up their assigned stations around Hector's coffin. Then they carried it, slowly passing members of his family, who stood as the procession reached their row. Each row, in turn, joined the procession until a line had formed, reaching all the way to the front of the church.

A Letter from Marcus

A few weeks after Hector's death, Marc gave everyone in his family a gift. He had written a letter to all of their children, he said, for the family to share with them whenever it was decided they were old enough to hear about HIV/AIDS. Hector's funeral had caused Marc to realize two things: that the kids needed information, and that he might not be around to talk to each and every one of them when they grew old enough.

Dear kids:

Hey, you guys, listen up. This is Marcus—your uncle, your big cousin . . . you know, Marcus. If I am still around when you get this, you can come ask me all the questions you want— just don't give me any attitude, because this is serious. And if I am not around to talk to . . . well, all I have to say is listen to your parents, especially when they read you this letter. Definitely do not give them attitude. They love you and are doing their job when they try to protect you, to help you grow up healthy so you'll live long enough to meet your own grandchildren. Yeah, I know that's not where your head is at now, but believe it or not, what you do with yourself now will help decide what kind of adult you'll become.

Do you want to look good and have fun? You have to be healthy. Do you want to be able to make money? You need your health. Do you want to live free? Then don't give yourself extra work by getting sick because you weren't careful with your body when you were young and thought nothing could hurt you. Do you want to live really free? Then don't take on extra responsibility and guilt because you might have made someone else sick.

Your body is yours to enjoy in the right way, at the right time, and with the right person. Your body is also yours to be responsible for, and responsible with. Grandma's genes are in you. She is a smart lady who has lived long and looked good doing it. She always thought twice before she did anything. And she always thought of others whenever she did anything.

I have to live with a disease for which there is no cure. I have to live looking at sadness in my beautiful wife's eyes. This sadness was planted before she even knew me, when I was in my teens. I went around having sex with people I didn't know, and they were having sex with people they didn't know. Some of those people were taking drugs with needles. I don't know who else got sick, but I did. I got HIV/AIDS, and I didn't even find out about it for years.

AIDS took its time taking over my body because I was healthy. It had to fight all the good health God gave me. Once I found out about it, I started fighting back, but it has been very difficult. I have to take multiple drugs every day. They make my stomach hurt. I can't eat whatever I want to, and I am not as good-looking as I used to be. My kids can see that their dad is sick. I am not the fun guy I want to be for them. I have to talk to them about things they are really too young to know about.

I thank God I am part of a big, caring family. I wouldn't even try if I had to go through this alone. But trust me, it hurts like hell to know you are making people you love sad. It is painful to know that you can't even live the few days you have left to the fullest. I'm begging you kids to appreciate what you have—life, health, and family—and take good care of it.

Run around playing soccer and basketball. Study hard. Learn extra things that are not even required. Put your youth and energy into helping others. Make good friends. Learn to play the guitar or do the latest dance. Double dutch. Or become a great cook like Grandma. Whatever. Just do it.

Be well. Be safe with yourself and with others. Build a good life.

Love,
Marcus

EPILOGUE

We have learned that not only can HIV/AIDS destroy a body, but it can also destroy a family, friendships, and even a community. We must learn not to stigmatize those who are afflicted, but to show compassion. Too many people walk away from those infected or, even worse, attack an individual by claiming that God has ordered this disease as punishment for their actions. But in reality, it is not God who has spread this disease, it is us. We should not allow it to interfere with God's mandate to love one another. Regardless of why they're suffering, we are called to be by their side in prayer and service.

There is one thing that HIV/AIDS cannot destroy: true love. The disease can grab the body and it might even grab the mind, but it cannot grab the soul. The soul belongs to God almighty and it is God's love that will always win the battle for the soul when individuals like you become God's agents and present God's greatest gift to those who are afflicted. This gift is the relief of burden and despair through Christ our lord. HIV/AIDS can *never* destroy God's love for the individual who suffers. Not only should our love be extended to any and all who are touched by HIV/AIDS, but also to the individual's family and friends. Many times I have been told of an HIV-infected person who has not been touched or held since being infected. The mental and spiritual anguish of being excluded from human relationships, in addition to having to confront one's ability to live, are sometimes too much for a person to handle and can lead to a depression that further debilitates the individual. I have been told countless times and know from experience that it is the sharing of God's love and the holding of hands through prayer or the joy of an *abrazo* (hug) that rejuvenates the spirit of an HIV/AIDS sufferer. It also does wonders for us who serve by providing us with a glimpse of God's true love, of the redemption of the spirit, and of the frailty of life. One cannot serve in this manner without being touched by God's spirit. Allow God to use you in this way and it will open new vistas into God's compassion and love.

What greater testimony can people of faith have than to be on the forefront of loving those who are afflicted? In the sacred scriptures (Matthew 25:31–46) Christ says that the positive we do for the hungry, the thirsty, the stranger, the naked, the sick or imprisoned, we do for Christ himself. Christ provides an opportunity for those seeking to be his representative.

So how can we join the HIV/AIDS struggle? It is clear that there are simple steps that we can take. Develop your spiritual side by putting yourself in the service of others. Find opportunities to educate others about HIV/AIDS. Be as ready as possible to be a friend and family member to those who might fall to the epidemic. Finally, fight against the disease. We have been asked by God to love our neighbor as we love ourselves. To love is to heal, whether it is through our good will, our prayers, or our acts of kindness. Join us!

For more information about this disease and how you can help, as well as additional resources available to you, please visit www.esperanza.us.

ACKNOWLEDGMENTS

I must first thank all the people who have participated in Pacto de Esperanza and to all the clergy who have been part of this effort for the last five years. To all the celebrities who gave their time to put together a CD and film, thank you. As with all ideas that come to fruition, I need to thank those who have helped and inspired me along the way. Thanks to Sheila Greco for her willingness to work with me. Many thanks to the Reverend Fred Estrada, to Dr. Ramón Gadea, executive director of Access Caribe, to the Reverend Rosa Caraballo, and to Nancy Rivera of Sembrando Flores in Miami. You are all frontline heroes in the battle against HIV/AIDS who were willing to share your experiences. *Gracias a todos.* Thanks to Miguel Gómez, director of OHAP at the U.S. Department of Health and Human Services, who read through the text and whose contributions are lifesaving. Special thanks to Dr.

Nils Kastberg, UNICEF regional director for Latin America and the Caribbean, for sharing with us the realities of the global epidemic.

I greatly admire and must thank the Atria team. My sincere appreciation goes to Judith Curr, publisher of Atria Books, who trusted an unpublished writer enough to move this series forward. Thanks to my editor, Johanna Castillo, for her great patience and for her willingness to continually challenge me. The rest of the team—Amy Tannenbaum, for her patience and support; Gary Urda, Michael Selleck, Sue Fleming, Christine Duplessis, and Melissa Quiñones—who have all contributed to this effort: Thank you.

APPENDIX:
HELPFUL ORGANIZATIONS
THROUGHOUT THE UNITED STATES

We hope that this book will be helpful in raising awareness about HIV/AIDS, and increasing participation in the efforts to prevent its spread. To that end, we provide a directory of organizations we have found to be actively engaged in research on HIV/AIDS, in providing assistance to those affected and their families, or in working in many other ways to prevent the spread of the virus. Many of the following organizations are specially dedicated to serving Hispanic communities, or at least have available Spanish-language resources and Spanish-speaking staff members and volunteers.

It is important to understand that every county health department clinic throughout the United States is required to have information and testing available. In addition, hospitals generally are required to provide HIV/AIDS services, including counseling and chaplains. These are particularly crucial in emergencies and crises, such as rape or other kinds of sexual abuse, when medical attention should always be sought.

We are pleased to note that many of the organizations actively involved in providing information, care, and support to those with HIV/AIDS are operated by people of faith. Nothing could be more consistent with true faith than to extend love and support to people who are ill.

HIV is still a real and present danger to public health worldwide, according to the United Nations' latest figures from its "AIDS Epidemic Update 2005." However, the report also carries the encouraging news that prevention efforts—where they have been put into place—are working. These efforts include the Caribbean nations, where a sudden and dramatic spread of the virus among women had initially caught leaders off guard. The percentages are still high, but this latest report indicates that the spread has been stabilized.

At this point in the pandemic, prevention is still much more effective than any treatment yet discovered. Following the release of the UN report, Lisa Power, head of policy at the Terrence Higgins Trust in the United Kingdom, said, "The global epidemic continues to grow. . . . Preventing HIV is far more effective than treating its aftermath."

We at Esperanza are committed to being part of the long-term solution, whether by supporting those who provide direct care, distributing information in the community, or keeping the issue of HIV/AIDS on the radar of public policy makers.

This appendix contains contact points where you can obtain more information on HIV/AIDS. (These resources can also be found via links on our website, www.esperanza.us.) If you seek help, I hope that one of these organizations can provide more information, direct medical help, and spiritual leadership and comfort. It is vitally important for you to understand, however, that if a group on this list fails you or approaches you in a way that makes you uncomfortable, you should move on to another group. There is an organization, a group, or a person that will address your question or need with the dignity you deserve. There is no question or need that is unimportant.

My personal prayer for you who have gone through this book is that God will keep you, watch over you, and use you as part of a growing family that will address members of this epidemic with the compassion, care, and love that God wants us to provide.

Bendiciones.

National Center for HIV, STD, and TB Prevention
Centers for Disease Control and Prevention (CDC)

Division of HIV/AIDS Prevention National AIDS Hotline:
National Center for HIV, STD, and AIDS Prevention, CDC
Mail Stop E-49
Atlanta, GA 30333
Phone: (800) 342-2437; for Spanish speakers, (800) 344-7432
TTY: (888) 232-6348
Websites: www.cdc.gov/hiv/dhap.htm
          www.cdc.gov

Several organizations we have closely worked with include the following.

Access Caribe Health Care Project

P.O. Box 195
Cheltenham, PA 19012
Founder: Dr. Ramón Gadea

E-mail: accesscaribe@juno.com

Access Caribe runs pilot projects aimed at improving public health throughout the Caribbean region.

Christian Community Health Fellowship

P.O. Box 23429

3555 West Ogden Avenue

Chicago, IL 60623

Phone: (773) 277-2243

E-mail: cchf@cchf.org

Website: www.cchf.org

The Christian Community Health Fellowship (CCHF) is a national network of Christian health professionals and others concerned about the health care needs of impoverished communities throughout the United States.

Esperanza Health Center

Parkview Medical Office Building, lower level

1331 East Wyoming Avenue

Philadelphia, PA 19124

Phone: (215) 831-1100

E-mail: dw.esperanzahealth@juno.com

Website: www.esperanzahealthcenter.org

Sembrando Flores

29355 South Federal Highway

Homestead, FL 33030

(305) 247-2438

Director: Nancy Rivera

Other important sources of information we can recommend include the following.

AEGIS (AIDS Education Global Information System): AEGIS offers up-to-date information and links with HIV/AIDS news sources from around the world, www.aegis.org.

The Body: A website of information on personal care and personal issues related to HIV and AIDS, www.thebody.com.

UNAIDS: The United Nations maintains regularly updated information on HIV/AIDS around the world on its UNAIDS website, www.unaids.org. The site is organized by region.

UNICEF: Specifically targets HIV/AIDS-related issues affecting women and children, an increasing concern in Latin America and around the world, www.unicef.org.

Kaiser Family Foundation

Headquarters:
2400 Sand Hill Road
Menlo Park, CA 94025
Phone: (650) 854-9400
Fax: (650) 854-4800
Website: www.kff.org

Washington, DC, office and Public Affairs Center:
1330 G Street NW
Washington, DC 20005
Phone: (202) 347-5270
Fax: (202) 347-5274
An important report, "Latinos and HIV/AIDS in the United States," may be found at www.kaisernetwork.org/health_cast.

Center for the Study of Latino Religion, University of Notre Dame

230 McKenna Hall

University of Notre Dame

Notre Dame, IN 46556

Phone: (574) 631-8831

Contact: Dr. Edwin Hernandez

The Center for the Study of Latino Religion created the report "Faith-based Responses to HIV/AIDS" (2004) on behalf of Esperanza USA. As part of the project, the research team compiled the following list of organizations that provide information, service, and advocacy.

Faith-Based Organizations

Chicago, Illinois area

AIDS Foundation of Chicago

411 South Wells, Suite 300

Chicago, IL 60607

Phone: (312) 922-2322

Website: www.aidschicago.org

AIDS Pastoral Care Network, Program of Access Community Health Network

1501 South California Avenue

Chicago, IL 60608

Phone: (773) 826-7751, (773) 257-6425

Bishop's Task Force on AIDS of the Greek Orthodox Diocese of Chicago

40 East Burton Place
Chicago, IL 60610
Phone: (312) 337-4130

CALOR, A Division of Anixter Center

3220 West Armitage, first floor
Chicago, IL 60647
Phone: (773) 235-3161
TDD: (773) 235-4039
Website: www.calor.org
Anixter Center website: www.anixter.org

Canticle Ministries

26 West 171 Roosevelt Road
P.O. Box 667
Wheaton, IL 60189-0667
Phone: (630) 588-9165

Jewish AIDS Network—Chicago

c/o Norman Sandfield
3150 North Sheridan Road, Apt. 10B
Chicago, IL 60657
Phone: (773) 275-2626
E-mail: norman@sandfield.org
Website: www.shalom6000.com/janc.htm

Prevention Partnership

5936 West Lake Street

Chicago, IL 60644-1833

Phone: (773) 378-4195

Website: www.preventionpartnership.org

New York City area

Catholic Charities, Diocese of Rockville Centre

Catholic Charities HIV/AIDS Services and Day Treatment Program:

333 North Main Street

Freeport, NY 11520

Phone: (516) 623-7400

Website: www.catholiccharities.com

Catholic Home Bureau

1011 First Avenue, seventh floor

New York, NY 10022

Phone: (212) 371-1000

Contact: Philip Georgini

E-mail: pgeorgini@chbureau.org

Website: www.catholichomebureau.org

Columbia Presbyterian Medical Center Pastoral Care

622 West 168 Street

New York, NY 10032

Phone: (212) 305-5817

Contact: Chaplain Raymond Lawrence

General Board of Global Ministries, United Methodist Church
475 Riverside Drive, Room 330
New York, NY 10115
Phone: (212) 870-3870
Fax: (212) 870-3624
Website: www.gbgm-umc.org

God's Love We Deliver
166 Avenue of the Americas
New York, NY 10013
Phone: (212) 294-8100
Executive Director: Nancy Mahon, Esq.
Website: www.glwd.org

Harlem Congregations for Community Improvement
2854 Frederick Douglass Boulevard
New York, NY 10039
Phone: (212) 283-5266
Website: www.hcci.org

Momentum Project
322 Eighth Avenue
New York, NY 10001
Phone: (212) 691-8100
Fax: (212) 691-2960
Contact: Rosalina Arocho
Website: www.momentumproject.org

Project Hope at New York Foundling Hospital
590 Avenue of the Americas
New York, NY 10011
Phone: (212) 633-9300, ext. 01
Contact: Janice Booker
Specialized foster boarding home care.

Philadelphia, Pennsylvania area

AIDS Mediation Project
Good Shepherd Neighborhood House Mediation Program
5356 Chew Avenue
Philadelphia, PA 19138
Phone: (215) 843-5413

**Archdiocese of Philadelphia Department for AIDS Ministry
Catholic Life and Formation Office AIDS Ministry**
Part of Catholic Life and Evangelization/Respect Life
222 North 17 Street
Philadelphia, PA 19103
Phone: (215) 587-3839
Contact: James Corr

Catholic Social Services
105 Prospect Avenue
West Grove, PA 19390
Phone: (610) 869-6500

Philadelphia Yearly Meeting of the Religious Society of Friends

1515 Cherry Street

Philadelphia, PA 19102

Contact: Raymond Bentman

Website: www.pym.org/pm/faith.php

Positive Effect Outreach Ministry (PEOM)

5815 Germantown Avenue

Philadelphia, PA 19144

Phone: (215) 848-6010

St. Luke's Hospitality Center for People with HIV/AIDS

Church of St. Luke and the Epiphany

330 South 13 Street

Philadelphia, PA 19107

Phone (church): (215) 732-1918

Phone (center): (215) 732-9346

St. Mary's Family Respite Center

3115 Spring Garden Street

Philadelphia, PA 19104

Phone: (215) 387-7730

Website: www.stmarysrespite.org

Siloam Ministries

1133 Spring Garden Street

Philadelphia, PA 19123

Phone: (215) 765-6633

Website: www.siloamministries.org

Los Angeles, California area

Minority AIDS Project (MAP)
Treatment Education and Advocacy Program
    5149 West Jefferson Boulevard
    Los Angeles, CA 90018
    Phone: (323) 936-4949

Project New Hope Episcopal AIDS Ministry
    340 North Madison Avenue, Suite 100
    Los Angeles, CA 90004
    Phone: (323) 665-2816
    Fax: (323) 665-2817
    Website: www.projectnewhope.org

El Proyecto del Barrio HIV Services
    8902 Woodman Avenue
    Arleta, CA 91331
    Phone: (818) 830-7033

Unity Fellowship Church Social Justice Ministries
    5148 West Jefferson Boulevard
    Los Angeles, CA 90016
    Phone: (323) 938-8322

West Hollywood Presbyterian Church
    7350 Sunset Boulevard
    Hollywood, CA 90046
    Phone: (323) 874-6646
    Executive Director: Reverend Dan Smith, Pastor
    Website: www.wehopres.org

Miami, Florida area

AIDS Ministries of South Miami-Dade

10735 Southwest 216 Street
Suite B-126
Goulds, FL 33190

Catholic Charities of the Archdiocese of Miami

HIV/AIDS Ministry
1881 Northeast 26 Street
Wilton Manors, FL 33305
Website: www.catholiccharitiesadm.org

Episcopal Diocese of Southeast Florida
Episcopal AIDS Ministry of Miami

Trinity Cathedral
464 Northeast 16 Street
Miami, FL 33133
Phone: (305) 373-0881, (305) 374-3372
Website: www.diosef.org

Plymouth Congregational Church, UCC

3400 Devon Road
Coconut Grove, FL 33133
Phone: (305) 444-6521
Website: www.plymouthmiami.com

National Organizations

ACRIA—AIDS Community Research Initiative of America

Website: www.acria.org

Website en español: www.acria.org/espanol

Agency for Healthcare Research and Quality—Advancing Excellence in Health Care—Minority Health

John M. Eisenberg Building

540 Gaither Road

Rockville, MD 20850

Phone: (301) 427-1200

Website: www.ahrq.gov

AIDS Action

1906 Sunderland Place NW

Washington, DC 20036

Phone: (202) 530-8030

Fax: (202) 530-8031

Website: www.aidsaction.org

American Red Cross Hispanic HIV/AIDS Program

American Red Cross National Headquarters

2025 East Street, NW

Washington, DC 20006

Phone: (202) 303-4498

Website: www.redcross.org/services/hss/hivaids/hispanic.html

Website en español: www.redcross.org/spanish

Latino Commission on AIDS

24 West 25 Street, ninth floor

New York, NY 10010

Phone: (212) 675-3288

Fax: (212) 675-3466

Website: www.latinoaids.org

Latinos Unidos Contra El SIDA (LUCES), Hispanic Federation

LUCES:

184 Wethersfield Avenue

Hartford, CT 06114

Phone: (860) 296-6400

Hispanic Federation:

130 William Street, ninth floor

New York, NY 10038

Phone: (212) 233-8955

HF hotline: (212) 732-HELP, or (212) 732-4357

Fax: (212) 233-8996

E-mail: info@hispanicfederation.org

Website: www.hispanicfederation.org

Lutheran AIDS Network

625 Fourth Avenue South, Suite 200

Minneapolis, MN 55415

Website: www.lutheranaids.net

"Stop, Think AIDS, and Go!": HIV/AIDS awareness game is to be found at the above website.

National AIDS Memorial Grove (NAMG)

856 Stanyan Street

San Francisco, CA 94117

Phone: (415) 750-8340

Toll-free: (888) 294-7683

Fax: (415) 750-0214

Website: www.aidsmemorial.org

National AIDS Memorial Grove (NAMG), a fifteen-acre site in San Francisco's Golden Gate Park, is dedicated to and memorializes those who have lost their lives to AIDS and also honors those who are currently living with HIV/AIDS (PLWAs). Volunteers are always needed to help with weeding, clearing, and planting the grove. A newsletter and hotline are available.

National AIDS Treatment Advocacy Project (NATAP)

580 Broadway, Suite 1010

New York, NY 10012-3295

Phone: (212) 219-0106

Toll-free: (888) 266-2827

Fax: (212) 219-8473

Website: www.natap.org

National Alliance for Hispanic Health
Community HIV/AIDS Technical Assistance Network (CHATAN)

1501 Sixteenth Street NW

Washington, DC 20036-1401

Phone: (202) 387-5000

Fax: (202) 797-4353

Hotlines: (800) 725-8312, (800) 504-7081

Website: www.hispanichealth.org

National Association of People with AIDS
> 8401 Colesville Road, Suite 750
> Silver Spring, MD 20910
> E-mail: info@napwa.org
> Website: www.napwa.org

National Council of La Raza, Institute for Hispanic Health (IHH)
> Corporate address:
> 1126 Sixteenth Street NW, sixth floor
> Washington, DC 20036
> Phone: (202) 785-1670
> Toll-free: (800) 311-6257
> Fax: (202) 772-1792
> Website: www.nclr.org

National Latina Health Network (NLHN)
> 2201 Wisconsin Avenue, Suite 340
> Washington, DC 20007
> Phone: (202) 965-9633
> Website: www.nlhn.net

National Latino Behavioral Health Association
> P.O. Box 387
> 506 Welch Street, Unit B
> Berthoud, CO 80513
> Phone: (970) 532-7210
> Executive Director: A. Marie Sanchez, BSW
> Website: www.nlbha.org/about.htm
> Global HIV Awareness Campaign
> Website: www.nlbha.org/resources.htm#globalhivawareness

National Minority AIDS Council
   1931 Thirteenth Street, NW
   Washington, DC 20009
   Phone: (202) 483-6622
   Website: www.nmac.org

Office of HIV/AIDS Policy (OHAP)
   200 Independence Avenue SW, Room 736E
   Washington, DC 20201
   Phone: (202) 690-5560
   Website: www.dhhs.gov (query for AIDS)

Office of Minority Health Resource Center (OMHRC)
   P.O. Box 37337
   Washington, DC 20013-7337
   Phone: (301) 251-1797
   Toll-free: (800) 444-6472
   TDD: (301) 251-1432
   Fax: (301) 251-2160

People of Color Against AIDS Network (POCAAN)
   Seattle Office:
   2200 Rainier Avenue South
   Seattle, WA 98144
   Phone: (206) 322-7061
   Fax: (206) 322-7204
   Website: www.pocaan.org

Prevención—Wellness Through Media

Prevención, Inc.

3057 Fourth Street NE

Washington, DC 20017

Phone: (202) 832-6789

Website: www.prevencion.org

Self Reliance Foundation (SRF)/Acceso Hispano, Hispanic Community Resource Helpline

529 Fourteenth Street NW, Suite 740

Washington, DC 20045-1700

Hispanic Resource Helpline: (800) 473-3003

Website: www.selfreliancefoundation.org

U.S. Department of Housing and Urban Development, Office of Community Planning and Development Office of HIV/AIDS Housing

451 Seventh Street SW, Room 7212

Washington, DC 20410-7000

Phone: (202) 708-1934

Website: www.hud.gov/offices/cpd/aidshousing

Website en español: http://espanol.hud.gov/offices/cpd/aidshousing

Regional Nonprofit Organizations

Eastern Region: New York City

Access Project/AIDS Treatment Data Network

611 Broadway, Suite 613

New York, NY 10012

Phone: (212) 260-8868

Website: www.atdn.org/index.html

Website en español: www.atdn.org/lared/index.html

Aid for AIDS

515 Greenwich Street, Suite 506

New York, NY 10013

(at Spring Street)

Phone: (212) 337-8043

Website: www.aidforaids.org

Alianza Dominicana/Hope Program

715 West 179 Street

New York, NY 10033

(between Broadway and Fort Washington Avenue)

Phone: (212) 795-4226

Website: www.alianzadom.org

Bailey House, Inc.

275 Seventh Avenue, twelfth floor

New York, NY 10001

(at West Twenty-fifth Street)

Phone: (212) 633-2500

Website: www.baileyhouse.org

Body Positive

19 Fulton Street, Suite 308B

New York, NY 10038

(at South Street Seaport)

Phone: (212) 566-7333

Website: www.bodypos.org

Bronx AIDS Services

540 East Fordham Road, second floor

Bronx, NY 10458

Phone: (718) 295-5605

Website: www.basnyc.org

Caribbean Women's Health Association

100 Parkside Avenue, fourth floor

Brooklyn, NY 11226

(between St. Paul Place and Parade Street)

Phone: (718) 826-2942, (718) 940-8386

Website: www.cwha.org

Coalition for Hispanic Family Services

Proyecto Familia

315 Wyckoff Avenue

Brooklyn, NY 11237

(between Gates and Linden Avenues)

Phone: (718) 497-6090

Website: www.hispanicfamilyservicesny.org

Community Healthcare Network (CHN)

Administrative Office:

79 Madison Avenue, sixth floor

New York, NY 10016

Phone: (212) 366-4500

Website: www.chnnyc.org

Community Resource Exchange

42 Broadway, twentieth floor

New York, NY 10006

Phone: (212) 894-3394

Website: www.crenyc.org

Gay Men's Health Crisis

Tisch Building

119 West 24 Street

New York, NY 10011

Phone: (212) 367-1000

Website: www.gmhc.org

Website en español: www.gmhc.org/espanol.html

Henry Street Settlement—Community Consultation Center

40 Montgomery Street

New York, NY 10002

(at Madison Street)

Phone: (212) 233-5032

Website: www.henrystreet.org

Hispanic AIDS Forum (HAF)

Website: www.hafnyc.org

Manhattan:
213 West 35 Street, twelfth floor
New York, NY 10001
Phone: (212) 563-4500

Queens:
62-07 Woodside Avenue, third floor
Woodside, NY 11377
Phone: (718) 803-2766

Bronx:
886 Westchester Avenue
Bronx, NY 10459
Phone: (718) 328-4188

HIV Law Project

15 Maiden Lane, eighteenth floor
New York, NY 10038
Phone: (212) 577-3001
Website: www.hivlawproject.org

Latino Commission on AIDS

24 West 25 Street, ninth floor
New York, NY 10010
Phone: (212) 675-3288
Fax: (212) 675-3466
Website: www.latinoaids.org

Minority Task Force on AIDS (MTFA)
123 West 115 Street
New York, NY 10026
Phone: (212) 663-7772, (212) 870-2691

New York City AIDS Housing Network
80A Fourth Avenue
Brooklyn, NY 11217
Phone: (718) 802-9540
Website: www.nycahn.org

Treatment for Life Center
Brookdale University Hospital and Medical Center
1 Brookdale Plaza, Aaron Pavilion, fifth floor
Brooklyn, NY 11212
Phone: (718) 240-5028

Eastern Region: Pennsylvania

Action AIDS
Website: www.actionaids.org

Center City Office:
1216 Arch Street, sixth floor
Philadelphia, PA 19107
Phone: (215) 981-0088; (215) 981-3365
Fax: (215) 387-7989

Washington West Project:
1201 Locust Street
Philadelphia, PA 19107
Phone: (215) 985-9206

North Philadelphia Office:
2641 North Sixth Street
Philadelphia, PA 19133
Phone: (215) 291-6111

West Philadelphia Office:
3901 Market Street
Philadelphia, PA 19104
Phone: (215) 387-6055

CHOICE/Community AIDS and Health Choices Hotline
1233 Locust Street, third floor
Philadelphia, PA 19107
Phone: (215) 985-3300
Website: www.choice-phila.org

Congreso de Latinos/Programa Esfuerzo
213 West Somerset
Philadelphia, PA 19133
Phone: (215) 763-8870
Website: www.congreso.net

Delaware Valley Community Health
Fairmount Primary Care Center
　　1412 Fairmount Avenue
　　Philadelphia, PA 19130
　　Phone: (215) 235-9600
　　Website: www.dvch.org

Latino Treatment Program
　　100 West Lehigh Avenue
　　Philadelphia, PA 19125
　　Phone: (215) 203-3000

Mazzoni Center
　　1201 Chestnut Street
　　Philadelphia, PA 19107
　　Phone: (215) 563-0652
　　Website: www.mazzonicenter.org

Philadelphia FIGHT
　　1233 Locust Street, fifth floor
　　Philadelphia, PA 19107
　　Phone: (215) 985-4851
　　Website: www.fight.org

Center for Minority Health, Graduate School of Public Health, University of Pittsburgh

125 Parran Hall

30 Desoto Street

Pittsburgh, PA 15261

Phone: (412) 624-5665

Stephen B. Thomas, Ph.D., Director, Center for Minority Health

Philip Hallen, Professor of Community Health and Social Justice, University of Pittsburgh

Website: www.cmh.pitt.edu

Eastern Region: North Carolina

Acción Hispana

AIDS Care Service

3 East Devonshire Street

Winston-Salem, NC 27127

Phone: (336) 723-6609

Fax: (336) 723-1863

Website: www.accionhispana.org

American Social Health Association

SALSA (STDs, Adolescents, and Latinos: Sexual Health Awareness)

Website: www.ashastd.org

Eastern Region: Washington, DC

Clínica del Pueblo, HIV/AIDS Department
2831 Fifteenth Street NW
Washington, DC 20009
Phone: (202) 462-4788
Website: www.lcdp.org

Lutheran Social Services of the National Capital Area
HIV/AIDS Services
4406 Georgia Avenue NW
Washington, DC 20011-7124
Phone: (202) 723-3000
Fax: (202) 723-3303
Website: www.lssnca.org

Washington AIDS Partnership
1400 Sixteenth Street NW, Suite 740
Washington, DC 20036
Phone: (202) 939-3379
Website: www.washingtonaidspartnership.org

Whitman-Walker Clinic
E-mail: latino@wwc.org
Website: www.wwc.org/latinoservices

Latino Services:
Phone: (202) 939-7881
Fax: (202) 939-1575
AIDS Information Line en español: (202) 328-0697

Administrative Facility:
1407 S Street, NW
Washington, DC 20009
Phone: (202) 797-3500

Eastern Region: Connecticut

Hispanic Health Council AIDS Unit (HHC)
175 Main Street
Hartford, CT 06106
Phone: (860) 527-0856
Website: www.hispanichealth.com

Hispanos Unidos Contra el SIDA/AIDS
116 Sherman Avenue, first floor
New Haven, CT 06511
Phone: (203) 781-0226

Latinos/as Contra SIDA
184 Wethersfield Avenue
Hartford, CT 06114
Phone: (860) 296-6400
Website: www.latinoscontrasida.org

Western Region: California

AIDS Project Los Angeles

Website: www.apla.org

APLA West
639 North Fairfax Avenue
Los Angeles, CA 90036
Phone: (213) 201-1639

David Geffen Center
611 South Kingsley Drive
Los Angeles, CA 90005
Phone: (213) 201-1600

Bienestar Human Services

4955 Sunset Boulevard
Los Angeles, CA 90027
Phone: (323) 660-9680
Website: www.bienestar.org

Bienestar Latino AIDS Project is a multiservice, multicenter agency, offering services in Los Angeles County, San Bernardino County, and San Diego.

Children Affected by AIDS Foundation

6033 West Century Boulevard, Suite 280
Los Angeles, CA 90045
Phone: (310) 258-0850
Website: www.caaf4kids.org

Clínica Para Las Américas
318 South Alvarado Street
Los Angeles, CA 90057
Phone: (213) 484-8434

El Centro Human Services
Milagros AIDS Project
2130 East First Street, Suite 350
Los Angeles, CA 90033
Phone: (323) 265-9228
Fax: (323) 265-7166

T.H.E. Clinic, Inc., Multiethnic HIV Prevention/Health Education Risk Reduction Program
Ruth Temple Health Center
3834 South Western Avenue
Los Angeles, CA 90062
Phone: (323) 295-6571
Fax: (323) 295-6577
E-mail: info@theclinicinc.org
Website: www.theclinicinc.org

Wall-Las Memorias Project
111 North Avenue 56
Los Angeles, CA 90042
Phone: (323) 257-1056
Website: www.thewalllasmemorias.org

Center for Aids Prevention Studies at the AIDS Research Institute, University of California, San Francisco
> 50 Beale Street, Suite 1300
> San Francisco, CA 94105
> Phone: (415) 597-9100
> Website: www.caps.ucsf.edu

Latino AIDS Project
> Instituto Familiar de la Raza
> 2639 Twenty-Fourth Street
> San Francisco, CA 94110
> Phone: (415) 647-4033

Latino Coalition for a Healthy California
> 1225 Eighth Street, Suite 500
> Sacramento, CA 95814
> Phone: (916) 448-3234
> Website: www.lchc.org

Mexican American Alcoholism Programs Incorporated
> Hispanic AIDS Community Education Resources (MAAP HACER)
> 4241 Florin Road, Suite 110
> Sacramento, CA 95823-2535
> Phone: (916) 394-2320
> Website: www.mapp.org
> Regions served include Sacramento and Yolo, California.

PACTO Latino AIDS Organization
  2876 Howard Avenue
  San Diego, CA 92138
  Phone: (619) 563-3622

Project Inform
  205 Thirteenth Street, Suite 2001
  San Francisco, CA 94103
  Phone: (415) 558-8669
  Treatment Hotline: (415) 558-9051
  Toll-free: (800) 822-7422
  Website: www.projectinform.org

San Francisco AIDS Foundation
  995 Market Street
  San Francisco, CA 94103
  Phone: (415) 581-7000
  Website: www.sfaf.org
  Website en español: www.sfaf.org/espanol.html

San Francisco General Hospital
San Francisco Area AIDS Education and Training Center (SFAETC)
National HIV Telephone Consultation Services

   995 Potrero Avenue
   Building 80, Ward 83, Room 314
   San Francisco, CA 94110-2859
   Phone: (415) 476-7070
   Toll-free: (800) 933-3413
   Fax: (415) 476-3454
   E-mail: bteague@nccc.ucsf.edu

Western Region: Nevada

AIDS Education Program/Nevada Hispanic Services

   Nevada Hispanic Services
   3905 Neil Road, Suite 2
   Reno, NV 89502
   Phone: (775) 826-1818

Western Region: Washington State

Pierce County AIDS Foundation (PCAF)

   625 Commerce Street, Suite 10
   Tacoma, WA 98402
   Phone: (253) 383-2565
   Website: www.piercecountyaids.org

Midwestern Region: Illinois

AidsCare

212 East Ohio Street, fifth floor
Chicago, IL 60611
Phone: (773) 935-4663
Website: www.aidscarechicago.org

Aids Legal Council of Chicago (ALCC)

188 West Randolph Street, Suite 2400
Chicago, IL 60601
Phone: (312) 427-8990
Website: www.aidslegal.com

Chicago House

1925 North Clybourn Street, Suite 401
Chicago, IL 60614
Phone: (773) 248-5200
Fax: (773) 248-5019
Website: www.chicagohouse.org

Children Affected by AIDS Foundation

Chicago Office:
70 East Lake Street, Suite 430
Chicago, IL 60601
Phone: (312) 580-1150
Website: www.caaf4kids.org

Howard Brown Health Center
4025 North Sheridan Road
Chicago, IL 60613
Phone: (773) 388-1600
Website: www.howardbrown.org/thecenter.asp

Midwest Hispanic Health Coalition (MHHC)
53 West Jackson Boulevard, Suite 628
Chicago, IL 60604
Phone: (312) 913-3001
Website: www.salud-latina.org

TASKFORCE AIDS Prevention
1130 South Wabash, Suite 404
Chicago, IL 60605
Phone: (312) 986-0661

Test Positive Aware Network
5537 North Broadway Street
Chicago, IL 60640-1405
Phone: (773) 989-9400
Website: www.tpan.com

Vital Bridges
Main Office:
348 North Ashland
Chicago, IL 60607
Phone: (773) 665-1000
Website: www.vitalbridges.org

Midwestern Region: Michigan

Julian Samora Research Institute, Research and Publications
Michigan State University

301 Nisbet Building

1407 South Harrison

East Lansing, MI 48823-5286

Phone: (517) 432-1317

Website: www.jsri.msu.edu

Midwestern Region: Minnesota

Chicanos Latinos Unidos En Servicio (CLUES)

2700 East Lake Street, Suite 1160

Minneapolis, MN 55406

Phone: (612) 871-0200

Fax: (612) 871-1058

Website: www.clues.org

Midwestern Region: Ohio

Cleveland Hispanic Urban Minority Alcoholism and Drug
Abuse Outreach Programs (UMADAOP)

Hispanic Community Services Coalition

3305 West 25 Street

Cleveland, OH 44109-1613

Phone: (216) 459-1222

Website: www.umadaops.com

Midwestern Region: Wisconsin

Minority HIV/AIDS Demonstration Project, Wisconsin Department of Public Health

Phone: (608) 267-2173

Website: www.dhfs.wisconsin.gov/aids-hiv

Mailing address:

Minority HIV/AIDS Demonstration Project

Division of Public Health

P.O. Box 2659

Madison, WI 53701-2659

Street address:

Minority Health Program, Division of Public Health

1 West Wilson

Madison, WI 53703

Southern Region: Florida

AIDS Project Florida, Community Health Care Center 1

2817 East Oakland Park Boulevard

Fort Lauderdale, FL 33306

Phone: (954) 537-4111

Website: www.chc1.org

Center for Positive Connections, Support and Resource Center

12570 Northeast 7 Avenue, Suite 104

North Miami, FL 33161

Phone: (305) 891-2066

Website: www.positiveconnections.org

Contact Care Resource

Administrative Office:

3510 Biscayne Boulevard, Suite 300

Miami, FL 33137

Phone: (305) 576-1234

Website: www.careresource.org

Hispanic AIDS Awareness Program/Programa de Informacion Sobre el SIDA (HAAP)

2350 Coral Way, Suite 301

Miami, FL 33145

Phone: (305) 860-0780

Website: www.emservices.com

League Against AIDS/Liga Contra SIDA

28 West Flagler Street, Suite 700

Miami, FL 33130

Phone: (305) 576-1000

Website: www.leagueagainstaids.org

Lock Towns Community Mental Health Center

HIV Prevention and Early Intervention Services

16555 Northwest 25 Avenue

Miami, FL 33055

Phone: (305) 620-4005

Website: www.fccmh.org

Miami-Dade County Health Department, Office of HIV/AIDS Services

   8600 Northwest Seventeenth Street, second floor
   Miami, FL 33126
   Phone: (305) 470-6999
   Website: www.dadehealth.org

South Beach AIDS Project (SoBAP)

   1234 Washington Avenue, Suite 200
   Miami Beach, FL 33139
   Phone: (305) 535-4733
   Website: www.sobeaids.org

South Florida AIDS Network (SFAN), Jackson Memorial Hospital

   1611 Northwest 12 Avenue, ACC East, first floor
   Miami, FL 33136
   Phone: (305) 585-5241

Union Positiva

   1901 Southwest First Street, third floor
   Miami, FL 33135
   Phone: (305) 644-0667
   Website: www.unionpositiva.org

SOURCES CITED

Caraballo, Reverend Rosa J., *Covenant of Hope/Pacto de Esperanza: A Woman's Healing Journey in the AIDS Epidemic*, ebed Press, Bronx, N.Y., 2004.

Esperanza USA and Center for the Study of Latino Religion, University of Notre Dame, *Faith-Based Responses to HIV/AIDS in the U.S. Latino Community: A Needs Assessment*, February 2005 (Edwin L. Hernández, Héctor Díaz, Rebecca Burwell, and Elizabeth Station).

Gadea, Ramón, and Daniel Lee, "The HIV Epidemic in the Caribbean: Access Caribe Project," *Health and Development: A Quarterly Journal of Christian Community Health Fellowship*, Vol. 25, No. 3, 2005.

Joint United Nations Programme on HIV/AIDS (UNAIDS), "Fact Sheet: Caribbean," 21 November 2005; 23 November 2004 (see www.unaids.org).

———, "Fact Sheet: Latin America," 21 November 2005; 23 November 2004.

———, "HIV Epidemic in India," 25 October 2005.

———, "Sub-Saharan Africa," 24 October 2005.

Joint United Nations Programme on HIV/AIDS (UNAIDS) and World Health Organization, "AIDS Epidemic Update 2005," 21 November 2005.

National Association of People with AIDS, "NAPWA Positive Voice Alert," 5 October 2005 (see www.napwa.org).

United Nations Children's Fund (UNICEF), *Children: The Missing Face of AIDS*, 2005.

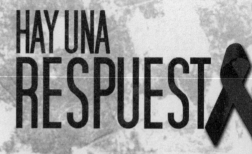

This DVD is available only in Spanish

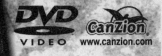

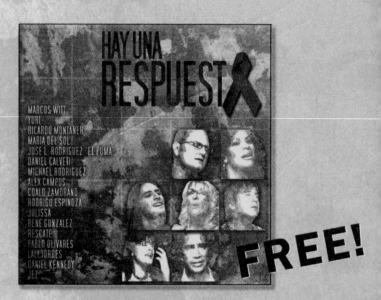
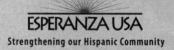